MUSCLE FUEL:

BALANCED RECIPES FOR

BUILDING MUSCLES

H. Y. Abraham

TESTIMONIES

Discover what others have to say about their experiences with "Muscle Fuel: Balanced Recipes for Building Muscles." These testimonials come from individuals who have embarked on their muscle-building journey with the help of this cookbook.

"I was struggling to find delicious and nutritious meals to support my workouts until I found 'Muscle Fuel.' The recipes are not only mouthwatering but also tailored for muscle growth. This cookbook has been a game-changer for my fitness journey."

- John D., Fitness Enthusiast

"As a vegetarian athlete, finding high-protein recipes can be a challenge. 'Muscle Fuel' not only offers an array of plant-based options but also makes them incredibly tasty. It's become my go-to resource for maintaining muscle on a plant-powered diet."

- Sarah V., Vegan Athlete

"I've always been intimidated by cooking, but 'Muscle Fuel' made it so easy! The step-by-step instructions and nutritional information are incredibly helpful. I've already seen improvements in my physique and energy levels."

- Michael P., Cooking Novice

"This cookbook is a treasure trove of delicious recipes that actually support muscle growth. The variety keeps me excited about my meals, and the expert tips have helped me fine-tune my diet for optimal results. Highly recommended!"

- Emily S., Fitness Enthusiast

"I've tried various diets and cookbooks, but 'Muscle Fuel' stands out for its focus on both taste and nutrition. The desserts section is a revelation! I never thought building muscle could be this enjoyable."

- Mark L., Sweet Tooth Connoisseur

"I've been following the meal plans and advice in 'Muscle Fuel' for a few months now, and I can see and feel the difference. The guidance on portion control and nutrient timing is spot on. This cookbook has become my fitness bible."

- Laura M., Dedicated Athlete

CONTENTS

ACKNOWLEDGMENTS

Creating this cookbook has been a labor of love, and I want to express my gratitude to the many individuals and sources of inspiration that have made this cookbook possible.

My Family and Friends

First and foremost, I want to thank my friends and family for their support throughout this journey. Your encouragement, patience, and willingness to be taste-testers have been invaluable.

Recipe Testers

To the dedicated individuals who volunteered as recipe testers, your feedback and enthusiasm have been instrumental in refining the recipes within this cookbook. Your taste buds and insights have helped ensure that every dish is both delicious and nutritious.

Nutrition and Fitness Experts

I extend my heartfelt thanks to the nutritionists, dietitians, and fitness experts who generously shared their knowledge and expertise. Your guidance has been pivotal in shaping the nutritional principles behind these recipes.

Photographers and Stylists

A special acknowledgment goes to the talented photographers and food stylists who brought the dishes in this cookbook to life. Your artistic flair and attention to detail have made the visuals as enticing as the flavors themselves.

Publishing Team

I am grateful to the dedicated professionals on the publishing team who transformed this project from an idea into a reality. Your expertise and commitment to quality have been instrumental in crafting a beautiful and informative cookbook.

Readers and Supporters

Last but certainly not least, I want to thank you, the readers and supporters of "Muscle Fuel." Your interest in this cookbook is a testament to the importance of combining health-conscious eating with the pursuit of physical well-being.

Every page of this cookbook is a reflection of the collective efforts and passion of everyone mentioned above. I hope "Muscle Fuel" inspires you to create nourishing meals that invigorate your journey toward a stronger, healthier you.

With heartfelt appreciation,

H. Y. Abraham

DEDICATION

This cookbook is dedicated to all those who believe in the transformative power of nutrition and the pursuit of a stronger, healthier self. It is for the individuals who understand that every meal is an opportunity to nourish their bodies and take a step closer to their fitness goals.

To the early risers and the late-night gym enthusiasts, to the novices and the seasoned athletes, to the home cooks and the culinary adventurers—this book is for you.

May these recipes not only fuel your muscles but also inspire your culinary creativity. May each dish be a reminder that strength and flavor can go hand in hand. And may every bite you take bring you closer to your vision of a healthier, happier you.

With dedication to your well-being and culinary delight,

H. Y. Abraham

DISCLAIMER

The information and recipes presented in this cookbook, are intended for general informational purposes only. While every effort has been made to ensure the accuracy of the content, the author and publisher do not claim to be licensed dietitians or healthcare professionals. Readers are advised to consult with a qualified healthcare provider or registered dietitian before making any significant dietary changes or embarking on a new fitness regimen.

The recipes in this cookbook have been carefully crafted with a focus on providing the nutrients necessary to support muscle building and overall well-being. However, individual dietary needs and preferences may differ. It is the responsibility of each reader to assess their unique dietary requirements and make informed choices based on their personal health and fitness goals.

The content of this cookbook is not intended to diagnose, treat, cure, or prevent any medical conditions. Any health-related information should not replace or be considered a substitute for professional medical advice or consultation. Readers are encouraged to seek guidance from qualified healthcare professionals for personalized dietary recommendations and fitness plans.

PREFACE

Welcome to "Muscle Fuel: Balanced Recipes for Building Muscles." I'm thrilled to embark on this culinary journey with you, and I'd like to take a moment to introduce myself and share the vision behind this cookbook.

The Importance of Nutrition in Muscle Building

We've all heard the phrase "You are what you eat," and when it comes to building muscle, this couldn't be truer. Proper nutrition is the cornerstone of any successful fitness journey. Whether you're an experienced bodybuilder or just beginning your path to a stronger you, the recipes in this cookbook are designed to support your muscle-building goals.

How to Use This Cookbook

"Muscle Fuel" is more than just a collection of recipes. It's your companion on the road to achieving your fitness aspirations. Here is how you can apply it.

- **Explore Diverse Recipes**: Dive into a diverse selection of recipes spanning breakfast, lunch, dinner, snacks, and desserts. Each dish has been carefully crafted to provide the nutrients your body needs to thrive.

- **Nutritional Information**: For your convenience, each recipe includes detailed nutritional information, making it easy to track your intake and meet your dietary goals.

- **Expert Advice and Tips**: Beyond recipes, find expert advice on nutrient timing, grocery shopping for muscle builders, portion control, adapting recipes to dietary preferences, and staying committed to your muscle-building journey.

- **Appendix**: Don't forget to explore the appendix, where you'll discover additional recipes, ingredient glossaries, cooking techniques, sample meal plans, and more.

"Muscle Fuel" is more than just a cookbook; it's your trusted resource for creating delicious, nourishing meals that align with your fitness goals. It's about quality over quantity, about savoring every bite while knowing that it's fueling your path to strength and well-being.

I'm excited to be part of your journey towards a stronger, healthier you. Let's get started and make every meal a step closer to your muscle-building aspirations.

With culinary enthusiasm and dedication to your success,

H. Y. Abraham

INTRODUCTION

In these pages, we embark on a journey to discover the delicious intersection of nutrition and strength—a journey that I'm excited to share with you.

About the Author

H. Y. Abraham is not just a cookbook author; they are a passionate advocate for the transformative power of nutrition. H. Y. Abraham has dedicated their life to understanding how food can fuel and fortify the human body.

Driven by a deep commitment to health and fitness, H. Y. Abraham embarked on a journey to explore the intricate connection between nutrition and muscle building.

Through "Muscle Fuel: Balanced Recipes for Building Muscles," H. Y. Abraham shares not only delicious recipes but also a wealth of knowledge on how to make every meal a step toward a stronger, healthier you. Their passion for quality, flavor, and results shines through in every dish, making this cookbook a trusted resource for individuals on their fitness journey.

With "Muscle Fuel," H. Y. Abraham invites you to discover the harmonious blend of quality nutrition and culinary delight, supporting your pursuit of strength and well-being, one meal at a time.

The Importance of Nutrition in Muscle Building

You've likely heard the phrase "You are what you eat." When it comes to building muscle, this couldn't be truer. Whether you're a seasoned bodybuilder or someone just starting their fitness journey, your nutrition plays a pivotal role in achieving your muscle-building goals.

Muscle growth isn't solely about lifting weights; it's about providing your body with the right nutrients at the right times. It's about understanding the role of protein, carbohydrates, healthy fats, vitamins, and minerals in supporting your pursuit of strength. It's about savoring every meal, knowing that it's a step closer to the healthier, more vibrant you that you're striving to become.

How to Use This Cookbook

"Muscle Fuel" is more than just a collection of recipes; it's a comprehensive guide to culinary excellence tailored to your fitness ambitions. Here's how you can make the most of it:

- **Explore Diverse Recipes**: Dive into a diverse selection of recipes spanning breakfast, lunch, dinner, snacks, and desserts. Each dish has been carefully crafted to provide the nutrients your body craves to thrive.

- **Nutritional Information**: For your convenience, each recipe includes detailed nutritional information, making it easy to track your intake and meet your dietary goals.

- **Expert Advice and Tips**: Beyond recipes, find expert advice on nutrient timing, grocery shopping for muscle builders, portion control, adapting recipes to dietary preferences, and staying committed to your muscle-building journey.

- **Appendix**: Don't forget to explore the appendix, where you'll discover additional recipes, ingredient glossaries, cooking techniques, sample meal plans, and more.

With this book you hold in your hands the keys to a world of culinary delights that support your fitness aspirations. These recipes are a celebration of quality over quantity, of flavor and nutrition working together in harmony.

So, let's embark on this culinary adventure together. Let's make every meal a step closer to your muscle-building aspirations.

With culinary enthusiasm and dedication to your success,

H. Y. Abraham

CHAPTER 1: BREAKFAST BOOSTERS

In the world of muscle building, breakfast isn't just another meal; it's the foundation of your day. The recipes in this chapter have been carefully crafted to provide you with the essential nutrients and energy needed to kickstart your morning and set the tone for a day of strength and vitality.

1.1. Protein-Packed Oatmeal

Ingredients:

- 1/2 cup rolled oats
- 1 cup milk (of your choice)
- 1/4 cup Greek yogurt
- 1 scoop of your favorite protein powder (unflavored or vanilla)
- 1 tablespoon honey or maple syrup
- 1/2 teaspoon vanilla extract
- A pinch of salt
- Toppings of your choice (e.g., sliced bananas, berries, nuts, seeds)

Instructions:

1. **Prepare the Oats:**

   - In a saucepan, combine the rolled oats and milk over medium heat. Stir well to prevent clumping.

2. **Simmer and Stir:**

   - Bring the mixture to a gentle simmer. Reduce heat to low and continue to cooking and stirring frequently. This will take about 5-7 minutes. The oats should absorb the liquid and become creamy.

3. **Add Protein Powder:**

   - After the oats are cooked to your desired level, remove the saucepan from heat. Stir in the protein powder, Greek yogurt, honey or maple syrup, vanilla extract, and a pinch of salt. Mix until everything is well combined.

4. **Serve and Customize:**

   - Pour your protein-packed oatmeal into a bowl. Now you are free to add your favorite toppings. Sliced bananas, fresh berries, chopped nuts, or seeds are excellent choices for added flavor and nutrition.

5. **Enjoy Your Protein-Packed Breakfast:**

   - Grab your spoon and dig in! This protein-packed oatmeal is not only delicious but also an ideal way to start your day with the nutrients your muscles crave.

Pro Tips:

- Adjust the sweetness to your liking by adding more or less honey or maple syrup.

- Experiment with different protein powder flavors to change up the taste of your oatmeal.

- For added texture and crunch, sprinkle some granola on top of your oatmeal before serving.

This Protein-Packed Oatmeal is more than just a morning meal; it's a muscle-building powerhouse. It provides you with a hearty serving of protein, slow-release carbohydrates, and essential nutrients to support your fitness goals.

Bright your morning with this delicious and nutritious breakfast!

1.2. Muscle-Building Breakfast Burrito

Ingredients:

- 2 large whole wheat tortillas

- 4 large eggs

- 1/4 cup diced bell peppers (any color)

- 1/4 cup diced onions

- 1/4 cup diced tomatoes

- 1/4 cup shredded cheddar cheese

- 1/4 cup cooked and diced lean turkey or chicken breast

- Salt and pepper, to taste

- Small amount of olive oil or Cooking spray

Instructions:

1. **Prepare the Eggs:**

   - In a bowl, whisk the eggs together until they are well beaten. Season with a pinch of pepper and salt.

2. **Sauté Veggies:**

   - Now heat a non-stick skillet over medium heat then lightly coat it with a cooking spray or small amount of olive oil. Add the onions and diced bell peppers to the skillet and sauté for 2-3 minutes until they start to soften.

3. **Add Eggs:**

   - Pour the beaten eggs into the skillet with the sautéed vegetables. Cook, stirring gently, until the eggs are just set but still slightly creamy. This should take about 2-3 minutes.

4. **Assemble the Burrito:**

- Lay out the whole wheat tortillas on clean surface. Divide the scrambled eggs evenly between the two tortillas, spreading them in the center.

5. **Add Toppings:**

- Layer the diced tomatoes, shredded cheddar cheese, and cooked diced turkey or chicken breast on top of the scrambled eggs.

6. **Fold and Roll:**

- To fold the burrito, first fold in the sides over the filling. Then, starting from the bottom, roll the tortilla up, tucking in the sides as you go.

7. **Serve or Grill (Optional):**

- You can serve the breakfast burrito as is or grill it in a hot, dry skillet for a couple of minutes on each side until it's lightly browned and crispy.

8. **Enjoy Your Muscle-Building Breakfast Burrito:**

- Slice the burrito in half diagonally if desired, and savor each bite of this protein-packed breakfast.

Pro Tips:

- Customize your burrito with additional ingredients like avocado, spinach, salsa, or hot sauce for extra flavor and nutrition.

- Prep the ingredients ahead of time to make morning assembly even quicker.

- This burrito is portable, making it an excellent choice for a busy morning or a post-workout meal on the go.

This Muscle-Building Breakfast Burrito combines protein, fiber, and essential nutrients in a delicious, easy-to-eat package. It's the perfect way to start your day and fuel your muscles for whatever challenges lie ahead!

1.3. Greek Yogurt Parfait

Ingredients:

- 1 cup Greek yogurt (flavored or plain)

- 1/2 cup granola (choose a high-protein, low-sugar variety)

- 1/2 cup fresh berries (blueberries, strawberries or raspberries)

- 1 tablespoon honey or maple syrup (optional, for added sweetness)

- 1/4 teaspoon vanilla extract (optional, for extra flavor)

Instructions:

1. **Layer the Greek Yogurt:**

- Begin by spooning a layer of Greek yogurt into a serving glass or bowl. The amount of yogurt you use will depend on the size of your container.

2. **Add the Granola:**

- Sprinkle a layer of granola on top of the yogurt. This adds a delightful crunch and extra protein to your parfait.

3. **Add Fresh Berries:**

- Next, add a layer of fresh berries. Berries not only add natural sweetness but also provide antioxidants and vitamins.

4. **Repeat Layers:**

- Repeat the layers by adding more yogurt, granola, and berries until your glass or bowl is filled to your liking.

5. **Drizzle with Honey (Optional):**

- If you prefer a touch of extra sweetness, drizzle honey or maple syrup over the top. You can also add a drop of vanilla extract for enhanced flavor.

6. **Serve and Enjoy:**

- Grab a spoon and enjoy your delicious Greek Yogurt Parfait. Each bite is a combination of creamy yogurt, crunchy granola, and the burst of flavors from fresh berries.

Pro Tips:

- Customize your parfait by using your favorite flavor of Greek yogurt or adding different fruits like sliced bananas or kiwi.

- To make your parfait even more protein-packed, consider using Greek yogurt with a higher protein content.

- Prepare these parfaits ahead of time in portable containers for a quick and nutritious grab-and-go breakfast.

This Greek Yogurt Parfait is a fantastic way to start your day with a protein punch and a burst of antioxidants from fresh berries. It's not only a delicious breakfast but also a smart choice for muscle recovery and sustained energy.

1.4. Scrambled Eggs with Spinach and Feta

Ingredients:

- 4 large eggs

- 1 cup fresh baby spinach, roughly chopped

- 1/4 cup crumbled feta cheese

- 1/4 cup diced red onion

- 1 tablespoon olive oil or cooking spray

- Salt and pepper, to taste

- Fresh herbs (e.g., chopped parsley or chives) for garnish (optional)

Instructions:

1. **Whisk the Eggs:**

   - In a bowl, whisk the four large eggs until they are well combined. Season with a pinch of salt and pepper.

2. **Sauté the Onion and Spinach:**

   - Heat a non-stick skillet over medium heat and add the olive oil or cooking spray. Once hot, add the diced red onion and sauté for about 2 minutes until they become translucent.

   - Add the chopped baby spinach to the skillet and cook for an additional 2 minutes, or until the spinach wilts and becomes tender. Stir occasionally.

3. **Add Eggs and Feta:**

   - Pour the whisked eggs into the skillet with the sautéed onion and spinach. Gently stir the mixture with a spatula to combine.

   - As the eggs begin to set, add the crumbled feta cheese. Continue to cook, stirring occasionally, until the eggs are cooked to your desired level of doneness. This should take about 3-4 minutes.

4. **Serve and Garnish:**

- Once the eggs are cooked to perfection, transfer the scrambled eggs with spinach and feta to a plate. If desired, garnish with fresh herbs like chopped parsley or chives.

5. **Enjoy Your Muscle-Building Breakfast:**

- Serve immediately and savor the creamy, cheesy, and protein-rich goodness of your Scrambled Eggs with Spinach and Feta.

Pro Tips:

- Customize your scrambled eggs by adding diced bell peppers, mushrooms, or tomatoes for added flavor and nutrition.

- Consider using low-fat or reduced-fat feta cheese if you're looking to reduce calorie and fat intake.

- For an extra protein boost, you can add a scoop of unflavored protein powder to the beaten eggs before cooking.

These Scrambled Eggs with Spinach and Feta are not only a delight to your taste buds but also a nutritious powerhouse for your muscles. Packed with protein, vitamins, and minerals, this breakfast will keep you energized and satisfied.

1.5. High-Protein Pancakes

Ingredients:

- 1 cup oat flour (you can make this by blending rolled oats)

- 1/4 cup protein powder (vanilla or unflavored)

- 1 teaspoon baking powder

- 1/4 teaspoon salt

- 2 large eggs

- 1 cup milk (of your choice)

- 1 tablespoon honey or maple syrup

- 1 teaspoon vanilla extract

- Cooking spray or a small amount of oil for the skillet

Instructions:

1. **Mix Dry Ingredients:**

   - In a mixing bowl, combine the oat flour, protein powder, baking powder, and salt. Mix them well to ensure even distribution of ingredients.

2. **Prepare Wet Ingredients:**

- In a separate bowl, whisk the two large eggs until they are well beaten. Then, add the milk, honey or maple syrup, and vanilla extract. Stir until everything is combined.

3. **Combine Wet and Dry:**

- Pour the wet ingredients into the bowl with the dry ingredients. Stir until you have a smooth pancake batter. If the batter is too thick, you can add a little more milk to achieve your desired consistency.

4. **Heat the Skillet:**

- Heat a non-stick skillet or griddle over medium heat. Lightly coat it with cooking spray or a small amount of oil.

5. **Cook the Pancakes:**

- Pour 1/4 cup of the pancake batter onto the hot skillet for each pancake. Use the back of a spoon to spread the batter into a round shape.

- Cook until you see bubbles forming on the surface and the edges start to set, usually about 2-3 minutes.

6. **Flip and Cook:**

- Carefully flip the pancakes using a spatula and cook for an additional 1-2 minutes on the other side until they're golden brown and cooked through.

7. **Serve and Enjoy:**

- Transfer your high-protein pancakes to a plate and serve them warm. Top with your favorite toppings like fresh berries, a drizzle of honey, or a dollop of Greek yogurt.

Pro Tips:

- Customize your pancakes by adding ingredients like mashed bananas, chopped nuts, or dark chocolate chips to the batter for extra flavor and texture.

- To keep the pancakes warm while cooking the batch, you can place them on a baking sheet in a preheated oven at a low temperature (around 200°F or 93°C).

These High-Protein Pancakes are a tasty and nutritious way to kickstart your day with the muscle-building power of protein. They're not only delicious but also a satisfying breakfast that will help you stay energized and focused on your fitness goals.

CHAPTER 2: LUNCHTIME POWER PLATES

In Chapter 2, we dive into the midday meal, transforming it into a powerhouse of nutrition and muscle-fueling goodness. These lunchtime recipes are designed to provide sustained energy, muscle recovery, and a satisfying break in your day.

2.1. Grilled Chicken Quinoa Bowl

Ingredients:

- 2 boneless, skinless chicken breasts

- 1 cup quinoa, rinsed and drained

- 2 cups water or chicken broth (for cooking quinoa)

- 2 cups mixed vegetables (e.g., broccoli, bell peppers, carrots), chopped

- 2 tablespoons olive oil

- 1 teaspoon garlic powder

- 1 teaspoon paprika

- Salt and pepper, to taste

- Fresh lemon wedges (optional, for serving)

- Fresh parsley or cilantro for garnish (optional)

Instructions:

1. **Prepare the Quinoa:**

   - In a medium saucepan, combine the rinsed quinoa and water or chicken broth. Bring to a boil, then reduce the heat to low, cover, and simmer for about 15-20 minutes or until the quinoa is fluffy and the liquid is absorbed. Remove from heat and fluff with a fork.

2. **Marinate the Chicken:**

   - In a bowl, combine olive oil, garlic powder, paprika, salt, and pepper. Place the chicken breasts in a resealable bag or shallow dish, and pour the marinade over them. Seal the bag or cover the dish and refrigerate for at least 30 minutes to marinate.

3. **Grill the Chicken:**

   - Preheat your grill to medium-high heat. Remove the chicken from the marinade and grill for about 6-8 minutes per side or until the internal temperature reaches 165°F (74°C) and the chicken is cooked through with grill marks. Remove from the grill and let it rest for a few minutes before slicing.

4. **Sauté the Vegetables:**

   - While the chicken is grilling, heat a tablespoon of olive oil in a skillet over medium heat. Add the chopped mixed vegetables and sauté for about 5-7 minutes until they are tender but still crisp. Season with a pinch of salt and pepper.

5. **Assemble the Quinoa Bowl:**

   - In serving bowls, divide the cooked quinoa evenly. Top with the grilled chicken slices and sautéed vegetables.

6. **Garnish and Serve:**

   - Garnish your Grilled Chicken Quinoa Bowl with fresh herbs like parsley or cilantro, and serve with optional lemon wedges for a burst of citrusy flavor.

Pro Tips:

- You can vary the vegetables based on your preferences or what's in season.

- For added protein, consider drizzling a bit of Greek yogurt or tahini dressing over the bowl.

This Grilled Chicken Quinoa Bowl is a balanced and protein-rich meal that's perfect for refueling during the day. Packed with lean protein, whole grains, and vibrant veggies, it's a satisfying and nutritious choice for lunch.

2.2. Chickpea and Spinach Salad

Ingredients:

For the Salad:

- 2 cups fresh baby spinach leaves

- 1 (15-ounce) can chickpeas, drained and rinsed

- 1 cup cherry tomatoes, halved

- 1/2 cucumber, diced

- 1/4 red onion, thinly sliced

- 1/4 cup crumbled feta cheese (optional, for added flavor)

- 1/4 cup chopped fresh parsley or cilantro (for garnish)

For the Dressing:

- 3 tablespoons extra-virgin olive oil

- 2 tablespoons fresh lemon juice

- 1 teaspoon Dijon mustard

- 1 clove garlic, minced

- Salt and pepper, to taste

Instructions:

Prepare the Dressing:

1. In a small bowl, whisk together the extra-virgin olive oil, fresh lemon juice, Dijon mustard, minced garlic, salt, and pepper. Set aside.

Assemble the Salad:

1. In a large salad bowl, add the fresh baby spinach leaves as the base.

2. Add the drained and rinsed chickpeas, halved cherry tomatoes, diced cucumber, and thinly sliced red onion on top of the spinach.

3. If desired, sprinkle crumbled feta cheese evenly over the salad ingredients.

Drizzle the Dressing:

1. Just before serving, drizzle the prepared dressing over the salad. Start with half the dressing and add more according to your taste.

Toss and Garnish:

1. Gently toss all the salad ingredients to coat them evenly with the dressing.

2. Garnish with freshly chopped parsley or cilantro for a burst of freshness.

Serve and Enjoy:

1. Serve your Chickpea and Spinach Salad as a light and nutritious lunch or a side dish. It's delicious on its own or alongside grilled chicken, salmon, or tofu.

Pro Tips:

- For a protein boost, consider adding grilled chicken breast, boiled eggs, or extra chickpeas to the salad.

- Customize the salad by adding olives, roasted red peppers, or your favorite vegetables.

This Chickpea and Spinach Salad is a delightful blend of fresh ingredients and zesty dressing, making it a perfect choice for a light and protein-packed lunch. It's a flavorful and satisfying addition to your muscle-building meal repertoire.

2.3. Turkey and Veggie Wrap

Ingredients:

For the Wrap:

- 2 whole wheat or whole grain tortillas

- 8 ounces lean turkey breast slices

- 1/2 avocado, thinly sliced

- 1 cup mixed greens (e.g., spinach, arugula, or lettuce)

- 1/2 cup cherry tomatoes, halved

- 1/4 cucumber, thinly sliced

- 1/4 red onion, thinly sliced

- 1/4 cup hummus (your choice of flavor)

- Salt and pepper, to taste

Instructions:

Prepare the Wrap:

1. Lay out two whole wheat or whole grain tortillas on a clean surface.

2. Spread a generous layer of hummus on each tortilla, leaving about an inch around the edges.

Assemble the Filling:

1. On each tortilla, place 4 ounces of lean turkey breast slices evenly down the center.

2. Add the thinly sliced avocado, mixed greens, cherry tomatoes, cucumber, and red onion on top of the turkey.

3. Season with a pinch of salt and pepper to taste.

Wrap it up:

1. To fold the wraps, first fold in the sides over the filling.

2. Starting from the bottom, roll the tortilla up tightly, tucking in the sides as you go. If needed, you can secure the wraps with toothpicks.

Slice and Serve:

1. Carefully slice each wrap in half diagonally.

2. Serve your Turkey and Veggie Wraps immediately or wrap them in foil for an on-the-go lunch.

Pro Tips:

- Customize your wraps with additional ingredients like roasted red peppers, shredded carrots, or your favorite veggies.

- Consider using flavored tortillas for an extra twist of taste.

These Turkey and Veggie Wraps are a convenient and protein-rich lunch option that combines lean turkey with a colorful assortment of vegetables. Packed with flavor and nutrients, they're perfect for a satisfying and muscle-building midday meal.

2.4. Salmon and Asparagus Foil Pack

Ingredients:

- 2 salmon fillets (about 6 ounces each)

- 1 bunch of fresh asparagus spears, trimmed

- 2 cloves garlic, minced

- 2 tablespoons olive oil

- 1 lemon, thinly sliced

- 1 teaspoon dried dill (or fresh if available)

- Salt and pepper, to taste

- Fresh dill or parsley for garnish (optional)

Instructions:

Preheat the Oven:

1. Preheat your oven to 375°F (190°C).

Prepare the Foil Packs:

1. Tear off two large pieces of aluminum foil, each about 12x18 inches in size.

2. Place half of the trimmed asparagus spears in the center of each piece of foil, creating a bed for the salmon.

Season and Layer:

1. Drizzle 1 tablespoon of olive oil over the asparagus on each foil piece.

2. Sprinkle minced garlic evenly over the asparagus.

3. Season both sides of the salmon fillets with salt, pepper, and dried dill. Place one salmon fillet on top of each bed of asparagus.

4. Lay two to three lemon slices on each salmon fillet.

Wrap and Seal:

1. Carefully fold the foil over the salmon and asparagus to create a packet. Seal the edges tightly to ensure the steam stays inside during cooking.

Bake in the Oven:

1. Place the foil packs on a baking sheet and transfer them to the preheated oven.

2. Bake for approximately 15-20 minutes or until the salmon is cooked through and flakes easily with a fork.

Serve and Garnish:

1. Carefully open the foil packs, being cautious of the hot steam.

2. Garnish the Salmon and Asparagus Foil Packs with fresh dill or parsley, if desired.

3. Serve your flavorful and nutritious foil pack directly in the foil or transfer it to a plate.

Pro Tips:

- You can customize your foil packs with your favorite seasonings, such as a drizzle of balsamic glaze or a sprinkle of red pepper flakes for some heat.

- For easy cleanup, consider using non-stick aluminum foil or parchment paper inside the foil packs.

These Salmon and Asparagus Foil Packs are not only delicious but also a simple and healthy way to prepare a complete meal in one packet. This dish is rich in protein, omega-3 fatty acids, and essential nutrients, making it an excellent choice for your muscle-building lunch.

2.5. Mediterranean Power Plate

Ingredients:

For the Plate:

- 6 ounces grilled lean protein (chicken, turkey, or tofu)

- 1 cup cooked quinoa

- 1 cup mixed greens (e.g., spinach, arugula, or lettuce)

- 1/2 cup cherry tomatoes, halved

- 1/2 cucumber, sliced

- 1/4 cup Kalamata olives, pitted

- 1/4 cup crumbled feta cheese (optional, for added flavor)

- Lemon wedges (for serving)

For the Dressing:

- 3 tablespoons extra-virgin olive oil

- 2 tablespoons fresh lemon juice

- 1 clove garlic, minced

- 1 teaspoon dried oregano (or fresh if available)

- Salt and pepper, to taste

Instructions:

Prepare the Dressing:

1. In a small bowl, whisk together the extra-virgin olive oil, fresh lemon juice, minced garlic, dried oregano, salt, and pepper. Set aside.

Assemble the Mediterranean Power Plate:

1. Start by placing a bed of mixed greens on each serving plate.

2. Add a scoop of cooked quinoa to the center of the greens.

3. Arrange the grilled lean protein of your choice (chicken, turkey, or tofu) on top of the quinoa.

4. Scatter halved cherry tomatoes, cucumber slices, Kalamata olives, and crumbled feta cheese (if using) around the plate.

Drizzle with Dressing:

1. Just before serving, drizzle the prepared dressing evenly over the entire plate.

Garnish and Serve:

1. Garnish your Mediterranean Power Plate with lemon wedges for a zesty finish.

2. Serve this nutritious and flavorful plate immediately and enjoy!

Pro Tips:

- Experiment with different lean protein options to keep your meals exciting and varied.

- For extra flavor, you can add a dollop of tzatziki or hummus to the plate.

This Mediterranean Power Plate is a vibrant and satisfying meal that combines lean protein, whole grains, and an array of Mediterranean flavors. It's a fantastic choice for a balanced and muscle-building lunch that will leave you feeling energized and nourished.

2.6. Veggie-Packed Quinoa Stuffed Peppers

Ingredients:

For the Stuffed Peppers:

- 4 large bell peppers (any color)

- 1 cup quinoa, rinsed and drained

- 2 cups water or vegetable broth (for cooking quinoa)

- 1 cup diced tomatoes (canned or fresh)

- 1 cup black beans, drained and rinsed

- 1 cup corn kernels (fresh, frozen, or canned)

- 1/2 cup diced red onion

- 1/2 cup shredded cheddar cheese (optional, for topping)

- Salt and pepper, to taste

- Fresh parsley or cilantro for garnish (optional)

For the Sauce:

- 1 (15-ounce) can tomato sauce

- 1 teaspoon chili powder

- 1/2 teaspoon ground cumin

- 1/2 teaspoon garlic powder

- Salt and pepper, to taste

Instructions:

Prepare the Quinoa:

1. In a medium saucepan, combine the rinsed quinoa and water or vegetable broth. Bring to a boil, then reduce the heat to low, cover, and simmer for about 15-20 minutes or until the quinoa is fluffy and the liquid is absorbed. Remove from heat and fluff with a fork.

Prepare the Sauce:

1. In a separate bowl, whisk together the tomato sauce, chili powder, ground cumin, garlic powder, salt, and pepper. Set aside.

Prepare the Peppers:

1. Preheat your oven to 375°F (190°C).

2. Cut the tops off the bell peppers and remove the seeds and membranes. Lightly season the inside of each pepper with a pinch of salt and pepper.

3. Place the hollowed-out peppers in a baking dish, standing upright.

Assemble the Filling:

1. In a large mixing bowl, combine the cooked quinoa, diced tomatoes, black beans, corn kernels, diced red onion, and half of the prepared sauce. Mix everything together until well combined.

2. Stuff each bell pepper with the quinoa and vegetable mixture, pressing down gently to pack the filling.

Bake in the Oven:

1. Pour the remaining sauce over the stuffed peppers.

2. Cover the baking dish with aluminum foil and bake in the preheated oven for 30-35 minutes or until the peppers are tender.

Add Cheese and Finish Baking (Optional):

1. If you're using shredded cheddar cheese, remove the foil after 30-35 minutes of baking and sprinkle the cheese evenly over the stuffed peppers.

2. Return the dish to the oven, uncovered, and bake for an additional 5-7 minutes or until the cheese is melted and bubbly.

Garnish and Serve:

1. Garnish your Veggie-Packed Quinoa Stuffed Peppers with fresh parsley or cilantro, if desired.

2. Serve these flavorful and nutrient-packed stuffed peppers as a hearty and satisfying meal.

Pro Tips:

- You can add other vegetables like chopped spinach, diced zucchini, or mushrooms to the quinoa filling for extra variety and nutrition.

- Customize the level of spiciness by adjusting the amount of chili powder to your taste.

These Veggie-Packed Quinoa Stuffed Peppers are a wholesome and delicious way to enjoy a variety of vegetables and whole grains in one meal. They are a fantastic choice for a muscle-building lunch that's both filling and flavorful.

2.7. Tofu and Broccoli Stir-Fry

Ingredients:

For the Stir-Fry:

- 14 ounces (about 400 grams) extra-firm tofu, cubed

- 2 cups broccoli florets

- 1 red bell pepper, thinly sliced

- 1 carrot, julienned or thinly sliced

- 1/2 cup snow peas, trimmed

- 1/4 cup sliced green onions

- 2 tablespoons sesame oil (for stir-frying)

- Sesame seeds, for garnish (optional)

For the Stir-Fry Sauce:

- 3 tablespoons soy sauce (low-sodium, if preferred)

- 2 tablespoons hoisin sauce

- 1 tablespoon rice vinegar

- 1 tablespoon honey or maple syrup

- 1 teaspoon freshly grated ginger

- 2 cloves garlic, minced

- Red pepper flakes (optional, for heat)

- Cornstarch slurry (1 tablespoon cornstarch mixed with 2 tablespoons water, to thicken sauce)

Instructions:

Prepare the Tofu:

1. Drain the tofu and place it on a clean kitchen towel or paper towels. Gently press to remove excess moisture. Cut the tofu into cubes and set aside.

Prepare the Sauce:

1. In a small bowl, whisk together the soy sauce, hoisin sauce, rice vinegar, honey or maple syrup, freshly grated ginger, minced garlic, and red pepper flakes if you desire some heat.

2. Prepare the cornstarch slurry by mixing 1 tablespoon of cornstarch with 2 tablespoons of water in a separate small bowl. Set both bowls aside.

Stir-Fry the Tofu:

1. Heat 1 tablespoon of sesame oil in a large skillet or wok over medium-high heat.

2. Add the cubed tofu and stir-fry for about 5-7 minutes, or until it becomes golden and slightly crispy on all sides. Remove the tofu from the skillet and set it aside.

Stir-Fry the Vegetables:

1. In the same skillet, add the remaining 1 tablespoon of sesame oil.

2. Add the broccoli florets, red bell pepper slices, julienned carrot, and snow peas. Stir-fry for about 4-5 minutes, or until the vegetables are tender-crisp.

Combine Tofu and Sauce:

1. Return the cooked tofu to the skillet with the stir-fried vegetables.

2. Pour the prepared stir-fry sauce over the tofu and vegetables.

3. Add the sliced green onions and mix everything together.

Thicken the Sauce:

1. Pour the cornstarch slurry into the skillet and stir well. Continue to cook for an additional 2-3 minutes, or until the sauce thickens and coats the tofu and vegetables.

Garnish and Serve:

1. Garnish your Tofu and Broccoli Stir-Fry with sesame seeds, if desired.

2. Serve this flavorful and protein-packed stir-fry hot, either on its own or over cooked brown rice or quinoa.

Pro Tips:

- You can add other vegetables like sliced mushrooms or water chestnuts for added texture and flavor.

- Adjust the level of spiciness by adding more or less red pepper flakes.

This Tofu and Broccoli Stir-Fry is a delicious and nutritious option for a muscle-building lunch. Packed with plant-based protein, fiber, and a variety of colorful vegetables, it's a tasty way to fuel your body and satisfy your taste buds.

2.8. Sweet Potato and Black Bean Bowl

Ingredients:

For the Bowl:

- 2 medium sweet potatoes, peeled and cubed

- 1 (15-ounce) can black beans, drained and rinsed

- 1 cup cooked quinoa

- 1 cup corn kernels (fresh, frozen, or canned)

- 1 red bell pepper, diced

- 1/4 cup chopped fresh cilantro or parsley (for garnish)

- Salt and pepper, to taste

For the Dressing:

- 3 tablespoons extra-virgin olive oil

- 2 tablespoons fresh lime juice

- 1 teaspoon ground cumin

- 1/2 teaspoon chili powder

- 1/2 teaspoon garlic powder

- Salt and pepper, to taste

Prepare the Sweet Potatoes:

1. Preheat your oven to 400°F (200°C).

2. In a large mixing bowl, toss the peeled and cubed sweet potatoes with a drizzle of olive oil, salt, and pepper until they are evenly coated.

3. Spread the sweet potatoes in a single layer on a baking sheet.

4. Roast in the preheated oven for about 20-25 minutes or until they are tender and lightly caramelized. Stir once or twice during cooking to ensure even roasting.

Prepare the Dressing:

1. In a small bowl, whisk together the extra-virgin olive oil, fresh lime juice, ground cumin, chili powder, garlic powder, salt, and pepper. Set aside.

Assemble the Bowl:

1. In serving bowls, divide the cooked quinoa evenly.

2. Add the roasted sweet potato cubes, drained and rinsed black beans, corn kernels, and diced red bell pepper on top of the quinoa.

Drizzle with Dressing:

1. Just before serving, drizzle the prepared dressing evenly over the ingredients in each bowl.

Garnish and Serve:

1. Garnish your Sweet Potato and Black Bean Bowl with freshly chopped cilantro or parsley.

2. Serve this nutrient-packed and vibrant bowl as a delicious and satisfying lunch or dinner.

Pro Tips:

- Customize your bowl with additional toppings like avocado slices, diced red onion, or shredded cheese.

- Feel free to add a protein source like grilled chicken, tofu, or shrimp for extra protein content.

This Sweet Potato and Black Bean Bowl is a wholesome and flavorful meal that combines the natural sweetness of roasted sweet potatoes with the hearty goodness of black beans and quinoa. It's a nutritious and muscle-building option that's both colorful and delicious.

2.9. Spinach and Mushroom Frittata

Ingredients:

- 8 large eggs

- 1 cup fresh spinach leaves, chopped

- 1 cup mushrooms, sliced

- 1/2 cup diced red onion

- 1/2 cup diced red bell pepper

- 1/2 cup shredded cheese (your choice of variety)

- 2 tablespoons olive oil

- 1 teaspoon dried thyme (or fresh if available)

- Salt and pepper, to taste

- Fresh parsley for garnish (optional)

Instructions:

Preheat the Oven:

1. Preheat your oven to 350°F (175°C).

Sauté the Vegetables:

1. Heat olive oil in an oven-safe skillet (cast iron works well) over medium heat.

2. Add the diced red onion and sliced mushrooms to the skillet. Sauté for about 5 minutes or until the mushrooms are tender and the onions are translucent.

3. Add the diced red bell pepper and continue to cook for another 2-3 minutes until the peppers are slightly softened.

Whisk the Eggs:

1. While the vegetables are sautéing, crack the eggs into a bowl and whisk them until well beaten. Season with salt, pepper, and dried thyme.

Assemble the Frittata:

1. Sprinkle the chopped fresh spinach evenly over the sautéed vegetables in the skillet.

2. Pour the beaten eggs over the vegetables and spinach.

3. Sprinkle the shredded cheese evenly over the top.

Cook on the Stovetop:

1. Cook on the stovetop over medium heat for about 5 minutes, or until the edges of the frittata begin to set.

Transfer to the Oven:

1. Transfer the skillet to the preheated oven and bake for approximately 12-15 minutes, or until the frittata is set in the center. You can check for doneness by inserting a knife or toothpick; it should come out clean when the frittata is cooked through.

Garnish and Serve:

1. Garnish your Spinach and Mushroom Frittata with fresh parsley, if desired.

2. Slice into wedges and serve hot. It's a delightful and protein-rich dish for breakfast, brunch, or any meal of the day.

Pro Tips:

- Customize your frittata with other vegetables like diced tomatoes, bell peppers, or zucchini.

- Experiment with different cheese varieties like cheddar, mozzarella, or feta for varied flavors.

This Spinach and Mushroom Frittata is a savory and nutritious dish that's packed with protein, vegetables, and flavor. It's a versatile addition to your muscle-building meal repertoire, perfect for any time you crave a satisfying and healthy meal.

2.10. Beef and Broccoli Rice Bowl

Ingredients:

For the Bowl:

- 8 ounces lean beef steak (such as flank steak), thinly sliced against the grain

- 2 cups broccoli florets

- 1 cup cooked brown rice

- 1/4 cup sliced green onions

- Sesame seeds, for garnish (optional)

- Sliced green onions, for garnish (optional)

For the Marinade:

- 3 tablespoons low-sodium soy sauce

- 2 tablespoons hoisin sauce

- 2 tablespoons rice vinegar

- 1 tablespoon honey or maple syrup

- 2 cloves garlic, minced

- 1 teaspoon freshly grated ginger

- Red pepper flakes (optional, for heat)

- Cornstarch slurry (1 tablespoon cornstarch mixed with 2 tablespoons water, to thicken sauce)

Instructions:

Prepare the Marinade:

1. In a bowl, whisk together the low-sodium soy sauce, hoisin sauce, rice vinegar, honey or maple syrup, minced garlic, freshly grated ginger, and red pepper flakes if you desire some heat.

2. Prepare the cornstarch slurry by mixing 1 tablespoon of cornstarch with 2 tablespoons of water in a separate small bowl. Set both bowls aside.

Stir-Fry the Beef:

1. In a large skillet or wok, heat a drizzle of oil over medium-high heat.

2. Add the thinly sliced beef to the skillet and stir-fry for about 2-3 minutes, or until it's browned and cooked to your desired level of doneness. Remove the beef from the skillet and set it aside.

Stir-Fry the Broccoli:

1. In the same skillet, add a bit more oil if needed.

2. Add the broccoli florets to the skillet and stir-fry for about 4-5 minutes, or until they are tender-crisp.

Combine Beef, Broccoli, and Sauce:

1. Return the cooked beef to the skillet with the stir-fried broccoli.

2. Pour the prepared marinade over the beef and broccoli.

3. Add the sliced green onions.

Thicken the Sauce:

1. Pour the cornstarch slurry into the skillet and stir well. Continue to cook for an additional 2-3 minutes, or until the sauce thickens and coats the beef and broccoli.

Serve Over Rice:

1. Divide the cooked brown rice into serving bowls.

2. Spoon the beef and broccoli mixture over the rice.

Garnish and Serve:

1. Garnish your Beef and Broccoli Rice Bowl with sesame seeds and additional sliced green onions, if desired.

2. Serve this delicious and protein-packed rice bowl hot and enjoy!

Pro Tips:

- You can use other cuts of beef like sirloin or ribeye for this recipe.

- Customize your bowl with added vegetables like bell peppers, snap peas, or carrots.

This Beef and Broccoli Rice Bowl is a savory and satisfying meal that combines tender beef, crisp broccoli, and a flavorful sauce. It's a fantastic choice for a muscle-building lunch or dinner that's both delicious and nutritious.

CHAPTER 3: DINNER DELIGHTS

3.1. Baked Salmon with Lemon-Dill Sauce

Ingredients:

For the Salmon:

- 4 salmon fillets (about 6 ounces each)

- 2 tablespoons olive oil

- 1 lemon, thinly sliced

- Salt and pepper, to taste

- Fresh dill sprigs, for garnish

For the Lemon-Dill Sauce:

- 1/2 cup Greek yogurt

- 1 tablespoon fresh lemon juice

- 1 teaspoon lemon zest

- 2 tablespoons fresh dill, chopped

- 1 clove garlic, minced

- Salt and pepper, to taste

Instructions:

Preheat the Oven:

1. Preheat your oven to 375°F (190°C).

Prepare the Salmon:

1. Place the salmon fillets on a baking sheet lined with parchment paper or lightly greased.

2. Drizzle each salmon fillet with olive oil and season with salt and pepper to taste.

3. Lay lemon slices on top of each salmon fillet.

Bake the Salmon:

1. Bake the salmon in the preheated oven for about 12-15 minutes, or until the salmon is cooked through and flakes easily with a fork.

Prepare the Lemon-Dill Sauce:

1. While the salmon is baking, prepare the lemon-dill sauce. In a bowl, combine the Greek yogurt, fresh lemon juice, lemon zest, chopped fresh dill, minced garlic, salt, and pepper. Mix until well combined.

Serve:

1. Once the salmon is done, remove it from the oven and transfer the fillets to serving plates.

2. Drizzle the prepared lemon-dill sauce generously over each salmon fillet.

3. Garnish with additional fresh dill sprigs.

4. Serve your Baked Salmon with Lemon-Dill Sauce with your choice of side dishes, such as steamed asparagus, quinoa, or a mixed green salad.

Pro Tips:

- Adjust the baking time depending on the thickness of your salmon fillets. Thicker fillets may need a few extra minutes in the oven.

- Customize the sauce with your preferred herbs and spices, such as parsley or chives.

This Baked Salmon with Lemon-Dill Sauce is a delightful and protein-rich dinner option that's both healthy and bursting with flavor. The creamy lemon-dill sauce complements the tender salmon perfectly, making it a delicious choice for muscle-building meals.

3.2. Lean Beef Stir-Fry

Ingredients:

For the Stir-Fry:

- 1 pound lean beef steak (such as sirloin or flank steak), thinly sliced

- 2 cups broccoli florets

- 1 red bell pepper, thinly sliced

- 1 cup snap peas, trimmed

- 1 carrot, julienned or thinly sliced

- 3 cloves garlic, minced

- 2 tablespoons vegetable oil (for stir-frying)

- Sesame seeds, for garnish (optional)

- Sliced green onions, for garnish (optional)

For the Stir-Fry Sauce:

- 1/4 cup low-sodium soy sauce

- 2 tablespoons oyster sauce

- 2 tablespoons rice vinegar

- 1 tablespoon honey or maple syrup

- 1 teaspoon freshly grated ginger

- 1/2 teaspoon red pepper flakes (adjust to taste)

- 1 tablespoon cornstarch mixed with 2 tablespoons water (cornstarch slurry, to thicken sauce)

Instructions:

Prepare the Stir-Fry Sauce:

1. In a bowl, whisk together the low-sodium soy sauce, oyster sauce, rice vinegar, honey or maple syrup, freshly grated ginger, and red pepper flakes. Set aside.

2. Prepare the cornstarch slurry by mixing 1 tablespoon of cornstarch with 2 tablespoons of water in a separate small bowl. Set both bowls aside.

Stir-Fry the Beef:

1. Heat 1 tablespoon of vegetable oil in a large skillet or wok over high heat.

2. Add the thinly sliced beef to the skillet and stir-fry for about 2-3 minutes, or until it's browned and cooked to your desired level of doneness. Remove the beef from the skillet and set it aside.

Stir-Fry the Vegetables:

1. In the same skillet, add the remaining 1 tablespoon of vegetable oil.

2. Add the minced garlic and stir-fry for about 30 seconds, or until fragrant.

3. Add the broccoli florets, red bell pepper slices, snap peas, and julienned carrot. Stir-fry for about 4-5 minutes, or until the vegetables are tender-crisp.

Combine Beef, Vegetables, and Sauce:

1. Return the cooked beef to the skillet with the stir-fried vegetables.

2. Pour the prepared stir-fry sauce over the beef and vegetables.

3. Add the cornstarch slurry to the skillet and stir well. Continue to cook for an additional 2-3 minutes, or until the sauce thickens and coats the beef and vegetables.

Garnish and Serve:

1. Garnish your Lean Beef Stir-Fry with sesame seeds and sliced green onions, if desired.

2. Serve this flavorful and protein-packed stir-fry hot over cooked brown rice or whole wheat noodles.

Pro Tips:

- Customize your stir-fry with additional vegetables like sliced mushrooms, water chestnuts, or baby corn.

- Adjust the level of spiciness by adding more or less red pepper flakes.

This Lean Beef Stir-Fry is a quick, tasty, and protein-rich dinner option that's perfect for muscle-building. Packed with colorful vegetables and a savory sauce, it's a balanced and satisfying meal.

3.3. Vegetarian Chili with Beans

Ingredients:

- 2 tablespoons olive oil

- 1 large onion, chopped

- 3 cloves garlic, minced

- 1 red bell pepper, diced

- 1 green bell pepper, diced

- 1 jalapeño pepper, seeded and minced (adjust to your spice preference)

- 1 zucchini, diced

- 1 cup corn kernels (fresh, frozen, or canned)

- 1 (15-ounce) can black beans, drained and rinsed

- 1 (15-ounce) can kidney beans, drained and rinsed

- 1 (28-ounce) can crushed tomatoes

- 2 cups vegetable broth

- 2 tablespoons chili powder

- 1 tablespoon ground cumin

- 1 teaspoon smoked paprika

- Salt and pepper, to taste

- Chopped fresh cilantro or green onions for garnish (optional)

- Shredded cheese and sour cream for serving (optional)

Instructions:

Sauté the Vegetables:

1. In a large pot or Dutch oven, heat the olive oil over medium heat.

2. Add the chopped onion and sauté for about 3-4 minutes, or until it becomes translucent.

3. Add the minced garlic, diced red and green bell peppers, minced jalapeño pepper, and diced zucchini. Sauté for an additional 5 minutes, or until the vegetables start to soften.

Add Beans and Corn:

1. Stir in the drained and rinsed black beans, kidney beans, and corn kernels.

Season and Simmer:

1. Add the crushed tomatoes, vegetable broth, chili powder, ground cumin, smoked paprika, salt, and pepper to the pot. Stir well to combine all the ingredients.

2. Bring the mixture to a boil, then reduce the heat to low. Cover and simmer for about 20-25 minutes, stirring occasionally.

Garnish and Serve:

1. Once the chili has simmered and the flavors have melded together, taste and adjust the seasoning as needed.

2. Serve your Vegetarian Chili with Beans hot, garnished with chopped fresh cilantro or green onions, and accompanied by optional toppings like shredded cheese and sour cream.

Pro Tips:

- Customize your chili by adding extra vegetables like diced carrots or celery.

- Adjust the level of spiciness by adding more or less chili powder and jalapeño pepper.

This Vegetarian Chili with Beans is a hearty and protein-packed dinner option that's perfect for muscle-building. It's a flavorful and comforting meal that's both nutritious and delicious.

3.4. Citrus-Marinated Grilled Chicken

Ingredients:

For the Marinade:

- 1/4 cup fresh orange juice

- 1/4 cup fresh lemon juice

- 1/4 cup fresh lime juice

- 3 tablespoons olive oil

- 2 cloves garlic, minced

- 1 teaspoon dried oregano

- 1 teaspoon dried thyme

- Salt and pepper, to taste

For the Chicken:

- 4 boneless, skinless chicken breasts (about 6 ounces each)

- Fresh orange, lemon, and lime slices for garnish (optional)

- Fresh parsley for garnish (optional)

Instructions:

Prepare the Marinade:

1. In a bowl, whisk together the fresh orange juice, fresh lemon juice, fresh lime juice, olive oil, minced garlic, dried oregano, dried thyme, salt, and pepper. This will be your flavorful marinade.

Marinate the Chicken:

1. Place the boneless, skinless chicken breasts in a shallow dish or a resealable plastic bag.

2. Pour the citrus marinade over the chicken, making sure each breast is well coated. Seal the bag (if using) or cover the dish, and refrigerate for at least 30 minutes to marinate. For even more flavor, marinate for up to 4 hours.

Preheat the Grill:

1. Preheat your grill to medium-high heat (about 375°F to 400°F or 190°C to 200°C).

Grill the Chicken:

1. Remove the chicken from the marinade and let any excess drip off.

2. Place the chicken breasts on the preheated grill and cook for approximately 6-8 minutes per side, or until they are fully cooked and have grill marks. The internal temperature of the chicken should reach 165°F (74°C).

Garnish and Serve:

1. Once the chicken is done, remove it from the grill and let it rest for a few minutes.

2. Garnish your Citrus-Marinated Grilled Chicken with fresh orange, lemon, and lime slices for a vibrant presentation.

3. Sprinkle with fresh parsley for an extra touch of color and flavor.

4. Serve your grilled chicken hot with your choice of side dishes, such as steamed vegetables, quinoa, or a fresh green salad.

Pro Tips:

- You can reserve a portion of the marinade before adding it to the chicken and use it as a flavorful sauce for drizzling over the grilled chicken when serving.

- For extra citrus flavor, consider adding some citrus zest to the marinade.

This Citrus-Marinated Grilled Chicken is a mouthwatering and protein-packed dinner option that's perfect for muscle-building. The combination of fresh citrus juices and aromatic herbs creates a delicious and refreshing dish.

3.5. Roasted Vegetable Quinoa Bowl

Ingredients:

For the Roasted Vegetables:

- 2 cups mixed vegetables (such as bell peppers, zucchini, cherry tomatoes, and red onion), diced

- 2 tablespoons olive oil

- 1 teaspoon dried oregano

- 1 teaspoon dried basil

- Salt and pepper, to taste

For the Quinoa:

- 1 cup quinoa, rinsed and drained

- 2 cups vegetable broth or water

- 1/2 teaspoon salt

For the Lemon-Tahini Dressing:

- 3 tablespoons tahini

- 2 tablespoons fresh lemon juice

- 1 clove garlic, minced

- 1/4 teaspoon ground cumin

- Salt and pepper, to taste

- Water, as needed for thinning

Optional Toppings:

- Fresh parsley or cilantro, chopped

- Crumbled feta cheese (for non-vegan option)

Instructions:

Roast the Vegetables:

1. Preheat your oven to 425°F (220°C).

2. In a large mixing bowl, toss the diced mixed vegetables with olive oil, dried oregano, dried basil, salt, and pepper until they are well coated.

3. Spread the seasoned vegetables in a single layer on a baking sheet.

4. Roast in the preheated oven for about 20-25 minutes, or until the vegetables are tender and slightly caramelized. Stir once or twice during cooking to ensure even roasting.

Prepare the Quinoa:

1. While the vegetables are roasting, prepare the quinoa. In a medium saucepan, combine the rinsed quinoa, vegetable broth or water, and salt. Bring to a boil.

2. Reduce the heat to low, cover, and simmer for about 15-20 minutes, or until the quinoa is cooked and the liquid is absorbed. Remove from heat and let it sit, covered, for 5 minutes. Fluff the quinoa with a fork.

Make the Lemon-Tahini Dressing:

1. In a small bowl, whisk together the tahini, fresh lemon juice, minced garlic, ground cumin, salt, and pepper. If the dressing is too thick, you can thin it with a bit of water until you achieve your desired consistency.

Assemble the Bowl:

1. Divide the cooked quinoa into serving bowls.

2. Top the quinoa with the roasted mixed vegetables.

3. Drizzle the Lemon-Tahini Dressing over the vegetables and quinoa.

Garnish and Serve:

1. Garnish your Roasted Vegetable Quinoa Bowl with fresh chopped parsley or cilantro.

2. If desired, sprinkle crumbled feta cheese over the top for a non-vegan option.

3. Serve this nutritious and protein-packed bowl hot, and enjoy the vibrant flavors.

Pro Tips:

- Feel free to customize your roasted vegetable selection with your favorite veggies.

- Add a protein source like grilled chicken or tofu for extra protein content.

This Roasted Vegetable Quinoa Bowl is a wholesome and satisfying dinner option that's packed with protein, fiber, and an array of colorful vegetables. The Lemon-Tahini Dressing adds a delightful burst of flavor.

CHAPTER 4: SNACKS FOR STRENGTH

4.1. Protein-Packed Smoothie

Ingredients:

- 1 cup unsweetened almond milk (or your preferred milk)

- 1 scoop (about 20-25 grams) of your favorite protein powder (whey, plant-based, or other)

- 1 ripe banana

- 1/2 cup Greek yogurt (plain or flavored)

- 1 tablespoon almond butter (or peanut butter)

- 1/2 teaspoon honey or maple syrup (optional, for added sweetness)

- 1/2 teaspoon vanilla extract

- 1 cup ice cubes (optional, for a colder and thicker smoothie)

- Fresh berries or sliced banana for garnish (optional)

Instructions:

Blend the Ingredients:

1. In a blender, combine the unsweetened almond milk, protein powder, ripe banana, Greek yogurt, almond butter (or peanut butter), honey or maple syrup (if using), and vanilla extract.

2. If you prefer a colder and thicker smoothie, add the ice cubes as well.

3. Blend all the ingredients on high speed until the mixture is smooth and creamy. If the consistency is too thick, you can add more almond milk to reach your desired thickness.

Garnish and Serve:

1. Pour your Protein-Packed Smoothie into a glass.

2. If desired, garnish with fresh berries or sliced banana for an extra touch of flavor and presentation.

3. Serve your delicious and protein-rich smoothie immediately as a satisfying and nutritious snack.

Pro Tips:

- Customize your smoothie by adding ingredients like spinach or kale for extra greens, chia seeds or flax seeds for added fiber, or a handful of oats for extra energy.

- Adjust the sweetness by adding more or less honey or maple syrup to suit your taste.

This Protein-Packed Smoothie is a quick and convenient snack option that's loaded with protein to support muscle growth and recovery. It's a delicious and versatile choice that can be tailored to your preferences with various add-ins and flavors.

4.2. Almond and Dark Chocolate Energy Bites

Ingredients:

- 1 cup rolled oats

- 1/2 cup almond butter

- 1/3 cup honey or maple syrup

- 1/4 cup unsweetened cocoa powder

- 1/4 cup ground flaxseed

- 1/4 cup chopped almonds

- 1/4 cup dark chocolate chips

- 1 teaspoon vanilla extract

- Pinch of salt

Instructions:

Prepare the Mixture:

1. In a large mixing bowl, combine the rolled oats, almond butter, honey or maple syrup, unsweetened cocoa powder, ground flaxseed, chopped almonds, dark chocolate chips, vanilla extract, and a pinch of salt.

2. Stir all the ingredients together until well combined. The mixture should be thick and sticky.

Shape into Bites:

1. Using clean hands or a cookie scoop, take small portions of the mixture and roll them into bite-sized balls. You can adjust the size to your preference.

2. Place the shaped energy bites on a parchment paper-lined tray or plate.

Chill and Set:

1. Place the tray of energy bites in the refrigerator for about 20-30 minutes. This helps them firm up and become easier to handle.

Store and Enjoy:

1. Once the energy bites have chilled and set, transfer them to an airtight container.

2. Store your Almond and Dark Chocolate Energy Bites in the refrigerator for longer freshness.

Pro Tips:

- Customize your energy bites by adding ingredients like shredded coconut, chia seeds, or dried fruits for variety.

- Feel free to use other nut or seed butters if you have preferences or allergies.

These Almond and Dark Chocolate Energy Bites are a fantastic snack option for refueling and providing a boost of energy. They are packed with wholesome ingredients like oats, almonds, and dark chocolate, making them both delicious and nutritious.

4.3. Cottage Cheese and Berries

Ingredients:

- 1 cup low-fat or fat-free cottage cheese

- 1 cup fresh mixed berries (such as strawberries, blueberries, and raspberries)

- 1 tablespoon honey or maple syrup (optional, for added sweetness)

- Fresh mint leaves for garnish (optional)

Instructions:

Prepare the Cottage Cheese and Berries:

1. In a serving bowl, spoon out the desired amount of low-fat or fat-free cottage cheese.

2. Wash and prepare your choice of fresh mixed berries. You can use strawberries, blueberries, raspberries, or any combination you prefer.

3. Arrange the fresh berries on top of the cottage cheese.

Drizzle with Sweetener (Optional):

1. If you'd like a touch of sweetness, drizzle honey or maple syrup over the cottage cheese and berries. Adjust the amount to your taste.

Garnish and Serve:

1. Optionally, garnish your Cottage Cheese and Berries with a few fresh mint leaves for a burst of color and flavor.

2. Serve this protein-rich and fruity snack immediately. It's a quick and wholesome option for satisfying your hunger and replenishing energy.

Pro Tips:

- Feel free to customize by adding a sprinkle of chopped nuts or seeds for extra texture and nutrients.

- Adjust the sweetness with your preferred sweetener or omit it altogether for a lower-sugar option.

This Cottage Cheese and Berries snack is an excellent choice for muscle-building, providing a balance of protein and antioxidants from the fresh berries. It's a refreshing and delightful snack that's both nutritious and delicious.

4.4. Hummus and Veggie Platter

Ingredients:

For the Hummus:

- 1 (15-ounce) can chickpeas (garbanzo beans), drained and rinsed

- 1/4 cup tahini

- 3 tablespoons fresh lemon juice

- 2 cloves garlic, minced

- 2 tablespoons olive oil, plus extra for drizzling

- 1/2 teaspoon ground cumin

- Salt and pepper, to taste

- Water, as needed for thinning

For the Veggie Platter:

- Assorted fresh vegetables for dipping (carrot sticks, cucumber slices, bell pepper strips, cherry tomatoes, etc.)

- Fresh parsley or cilantro for garnish (optional)

Instructions:

Prepare the Hummus:

1. In a food processor, combine the drained and rinsed chickpeas, tahini, fresh lemon juice, minced garlic, olive oil, ground cumin, salt, and pepper.

2. Blend the ingredients until smooth. If the mixture is too thick, you can add a little water, one tablespoon at a time, until you reach your desired consistency.

Assemble the Veggie Platter:

1. Wash and prepare an assortment of fresh vegetables for dipping. Popular choices include carrot sticks, cucumber slices, bell pepper strips, cherry tomatoes, and more. Use your favorites or whatever is in season.

2. Arrange the freshly cut vegetables on a platter.

Serve:

1. Transfer the homemade hummus to a serving bowl.

2. Optionally, drizzle a bit of olive oil on top of the hummus and garnish with fresh parsley or cilantro for added flavor and presentation.

3. Place the bowl of hummus in the center of the veggie platter.

4. Serve your Hummus and Veggie Platter as a wholesome and protein-rich snack or appetizer. Encourage dipping and enjoying the combination of creamy hummus and crisp, fresh vegetables.

Pro Tips:

- Customize your hummus with additional ingredients like roasted red peppers, sun-dried tomatoes, or smoked paprika for unique flavors.

- Add a sprinkle of paprika or a dash of hot sauce for extra zing.

This Hummus and Veggie Platter is a nutritious and satisfying snack option that combines the creaminess of homemade hummus with the freshness of assorted vegetables. It's a great choice for fueling your muscles and providing essential nutrients.

4.5. Nut Butter Banana Toast

Ingredients:

- 2 slices of whole-grain bread (or your preferred bread)

- 2 tablespoons of your favorite nut butter (peanut butter, almond butter, or any nut butter of choice)

- 1 ripe banana, thinly sliced

- 1 teaspoon honey or maple syrup (optional, for added sweetness)

- Pinch of cinnamon (optional, for extra flavor)

- Chopped nuts or seeds for garnish (optional)

Instructions:

Toast the Bread:

1. Toast the two slices of whole-grain bread until they reach your desired level of crispiness.

Spread Nut Butter:

1. While the bread is still warm, spread one tablespoon of your chosen nut butter on each slice of toasted bread. Ensure an even layer.

Add Banana Slices:

1. Arrange the thinly sliced banana over the nut butter on each piece of toast.

Drizzle with Sweetener (Optional):

1. If you prefer a touch of sweetness, drizzle honey or maple syrup over the banana slices. Adjust the amount to your taste.

Sprinkle with Cinnamon (Optional):

1. For an extra burst of flavor, sprinkle a pinch of cinnamon over the banana slices.

Garnish (Optional):

1. Optionally, garnish your Nut Butter Banana Toast with chopped nuts or seeds for added texture and nutrition.

Serve:

1. Serve your Nut Butter Banana Toast immediately as a satisfying and protein-rich snack or quick breakfast option.

Pro Tips:

- Experiment with different nut butters and bread varieties to discover your favorite flavor combinations.

- For a twist, consider adding a sprinkle of chia seeds or flax seeds for extra fiber and nutrients.

This Nut Butter Banana Toast is a straightforward yet delicious snack that provides a balance of protein, healthy fats, and carbohydrates—perfect for muscle recovery and energy replenishment. It's a versatile option that can be enjoyed any time of day.

CHAPTER 5: DESSERTS WITH A TWIST

In this chapter, we're exploring desserts that not only satisfy your sweet tooth but also contribute to your muscle-building goals. These treats are packed with wholesome ingredients and creative twists to make your post-workout indulgence guilt-free.

5.1. Protein-Packed Chocolate Avocado Mousse

Ingredients:

- 2 ripe avocados, peeled and pitted

- 1/4 cup unsweetened cocoa powder

- 1/4 cup your choice of protein powder (chocolate-flavored or plain)

- 1/4 cup honey or maple syrup (adjust to your preferred level of sweetness)

- 1 teaspoon vanilla extract

- A pinch of salt

- Fresh berries and chopped nuts for garnish (optional)

Instructions:

Blend the Avocado Base:

1. In a food processor or blender, combine the ripe avocados, unsweetened cocoa powder, protein powder, honey or maple syrup, vanilla extract, and a pinch of salt.

2. Blend the ingredients until you achieve a smooth and creamy mousse-like consistency. You may need to stop and scrape down the sides to ensure everything is well combined.

Taste and Adjust:

1. Taste the chocolate avocado mousse and adjust the sweetness or thickness as needed. Add more honey or maple syrup for sweetness or a splash of milk (dairy or plant-based) for a smoother consistency.

Chill and Serve:

1. Transfer the chocolate avocado mousse into serving bowls or glasses.

2. Cover and refrigerate for at least 30 minutes to allow the mousse to chill and set.

Garnish and Enjoy:

1. When ready to serve, garnish your Protein-Packed Chocolate Avocado Mousse with fresh berries and chopped nuts for added texture and flavor.

2. Serve this protein-rich and chocolaty dessert to satisfy your sweet tooth while supporting your muscle-building goals.

Pro Tips:

- Customize the mousse by adding a touch of cinnamon or a sprinkle of sea salt for extra depth of flavor.

- Experiment with different protein powders to find your favorite flavor combination.

This Protein-Packed Chocolate Avocado Mousse is a delightful and nutritious dessert option that combines the richness of avocados with the goodness of chocolate and protein. It's a satisfying treat that supports your muscle recovery efforts.

5.2. Baked Apple with Greek Yogurt and Cinnamon

Ingredients:

- 2 apples (such as Granny Smith or Honeycrisp)

- 1/2 cup Greek yogurt (plain or vanilla)

- 1 tablespoon honey or maple syrup

- 1/2 teaspoon ground cinnamon

- 1/4 teaspoon nutmeg (optional)

- Chopped nuts (such as walnuts or almonds) for garnish (optional)

- Raisins or dried cranberries for garnish (optional)

Instructions:

Prepare the Apples:

1. Preheat your oven to 350°F (175°C).

2. Wash the apples and carefully remove the core, creating a well in the center but leaving the bottom intact. You can use an apple corer or a sharp knife to do this.

3. Place the cored apples in a baking dish.

Mix the Filling:

1. In a small bowl, combine the Greek yogurt, honey or maple syrup, ground cinnamon, and nutmeg (if using). Stir until the mixture is well blended.

Fill the Apples:

1. Spoon the yogurt mixture into the center well of each apple, filling it generously.

Bake the Apples:

1. Cover the baking dish with foil and place it in the preheated oven.

2. Bake for about 25-30 minutes, or until the apples are tender and can be easily pierced with a fork.

Garnish and Serve:

1. Once the baked apples are done, remove them from the oven.

2. Garnish your Baked Apple with Greek Yogurt and Cinnamon with chopped nuts and raisins or dried cranberries for added flavor and texture.

3. Serve your warm and comforting dessert immediately. It's a wholesome treat that satisfies your sweet cravings while providing protein and essential nutrients.

Pro Tips:

- Customize the filling by adding a dash of vanilla extract or a sprinkle of brown sugar for extra sweetness.

- Experiment with different nuts and dried fruits for unique variations.

This Baked Apple with Greek Yogurt and Cinnamon is a delightful and nutritious dessert option that celebrates the natural sweetness of apples while adding creaminess and flavor with Greek yogurt. It's a comforting treat that aligns perfectly with your muscle-building journey.

5.3. Protein-Packed Fruit Salad

Ingredients:

For the Salad:

- 2 cups mixed fresh berries (such as strawberries, blueberries, raspberries)

- 1 cup diced mango

- 1 cup diced pineapple

- 1/2 cup diced kiwi

- 1/2 cup diced cantaloupe or honeydew melon

- 1/4 cup pomegranate seeds (optional)

- 1/4 cup chopped nuts (such as almonds or walnuts)

- 2 tablespoons chia seeds (optional)

For the Protein Boost:

- 1 scoop of your favorite protein powder (vanilla or berry-flavored)

- 1/4 cup water (adjust as needed)

For the Dressing:

- 2 tablespoons fresh lime juice

- 1 tablespoon honey or maple syrup (adjust to your preferred level of sweetness)

- Fresh mint leaves for garnish (optional)

Instructions:

Prepare the Fruit:

1. Wash, peel, and dice the mango, pineapple, kiwi, cantaloupe or honeydew melon, and any other fruits you're using. Place them in a large mixing bowl.

2. Add the mixed fresh berries, pomegranate seeds (if using), and chopped nuts to the bowl.

3. Optionally, sprinkle chia seeds over the fruit for added texture and nutrients.

Mix the Protein Boost:

1. In a separate bowl, mix the protein powder with water until it forms a smooth, protein-rich liquid. Adjust the water amount as needed to achieve your desired consistency.

Dress the Salad:

1. Drizzle the fresh lime juice and honey or maple syrup (for sweetness) over the prepared fruit in the mixing bowl.

2. Pour the protein boost mixture over the fruit as well.

3. Gently toss all the ingredients together until the fruit is evenly coated with the dressing and protein boost.

Chill and Serve:

1. Cover the bowl and refrigerate the Protein-Packed Fruit Salad for about 15-20 minutes to allow the flavors to meld and the salad to chill slightly.

Garnish and Enjoy:

1. When ready to serve, garnish your Protein-Packed Fruit Salad with fresh mint leaves for a burst of freshness and presentation.

2. Serve this colorful and protein-rich fruit salad as a delicious and nutritious dessert or post-workout snack that supports your muscle-building journey.

Pro Tips:

- Customize your fruit selection based on what's in season or your personal preferences.

- Experiment with different flavors of protein powder to create unique variations of this salad.

This Protein-Packed Fruit Salad is a refreshing and wholesome dessert that's packed with antioxidants, fiber, and protein. It's a delightful way to satisfy your sweet tooth while nourishing your muscles.

5.4. Peanut Butter Banana Ice Cream

Ingredients:

- 4 ripe bananas, peeled, sliced, and frozen

- 2 tablespoons smooth peanut butter (unsalted)

- 1 teaspoon honey or maple syrup (optional, for added sweetness)

- 1/4 teaspoon vanilla extract

- A pinch of salt

- Chopped peanuts or chocolate chips for garnish (optional)

Instructions:

Prepare the Frozen Bananas:

1. Start by slicing ripe bananas into coins and placing them in a single layer on a parchment paper-lined tray or plate.

2. Freeze the banana slices for at least 2-3 hours or until they are completely frozen.

Blend the Ice Cream:

1. Once the banana slices are frozen solid, transfer them to a blender or food processor.

2. Add the smooth peanut butter, honey or maple syrup (if using), vanilla extract, and a pinch of salt to the blender.

3. Blend all the ingredients until you achieve a creamy and smooth ice cream consistency. You may need to stop and scrape down the sides to ensure thorough blending.

Taste and Adjust:

1. Taste the peanut butter banana ice cream and adjust the sweetness or peanut butter flavor to your liking. Add more honey, maple syrup, or peanut butter if desired.

Serve:

1. Transfer the freshly made Peanut Butter Banana Ice Cream to serving bowls.

2. Optionally, garnish with chopped peanuts or chocolate chips for added texture and flavor.

3. Serve your homemade ice cream immediately as a guilt-free and protein-rich dessert that satisfies your cravings.

Pro Tips:

- For a twist, you can add a sprinkle of cinnamon or a drizzle of chocolate sauce on top.

- Experiment with different nut or seed butters for unique flavors.

This Peanut Butter Banana Ice Cream is a delightful and wholesome dessert that mimics the creaminess of traditional ice cream without any dairy. It's an excellent choice for satisfying your sweet tooth while supporting your muscle-building journey.

5.5. Greek Yogurt Berry Parfait

Ingredients:

- 1 cup Greek yogurt (plain or vanilla)

- 1 cup mixed fresh berries (such as strawberries, blueberries, raspberries)

- 1 tablespoon honey or maple syrup (adjust to your preferred level of sweetness)

- 1/4 cup granola (your choice of flavor)

- Fresh mint leaves for garnish (optional)

Instructions:

Prepare the Greek Yogurt Layer:

1. In a bowl, combine the Greek yogurt and honey or maple syrup. Stir until the sweetener is evenly mixed into the yogurt. Adjust the sweetness to your liking.

Assemble the Parfait:

1. In serving glasses or bowls, start by adding a spoonful of the sweetened Greek yogurt at the bottom.

2. Add a layer of mixed fresh berries on top of the yogurt.

3. Sprinkle a layer of granola over the berries. You can use your favorite granola flavor for variety.

Repeat the Layers:

1. Repeat the layers as desired, adding more yogurt, berries, and granola until the glass is filled.

Garnish and Serve:

1. Optionally, garnish your Greek Yogurt Berry Parfait with fresh mint leaves for a burst of color and flavor.

2. Serve this visually appealing and protein-rich dessert immediately as a delightful way to satisfy your sweet tooth while supporting your muscle-building goals.

Pro Tips:

- Customize your parfait by adding a drizzle of nut butter or a sprinkle of chia seeds for extra nutrition and flavor.

- Experiment with different types of yogurt or dairy-free alternatives for dietary preferences.

This Greek Yogurt Berry Parfait is a refreshing and nutritious dessert option that combines the creaminess of Greek yogurt with the sweetness of fresh berries and the crunch of granola. It's a perfect treat to enjoy any time of day while fueling your muscles.

5.6. Chocolate Protein Bites

Ingredients:

- 1 cup rolled oats

- 1/2 cup chocolate protein powder

- 1/4 cup natural peanut butter (or any nut/seed butter of choice)

- 1/4 cup honey or maple syrup

- 1/4 cup dark chocolate chips

- 1 teaspoon vanilla extract

- A pinch of salt

Instructions:

Prepare the Mixture:

1. In a mixing bowl, combine the rolled oats, chocolate protein powder, natural peanut butter, honey or maple syrup, dark chocolate chips, vanilla extract, and a pinch of salt.

2. Stir all the ingredients together until the mixture is well combined. It should be sticky and hold together.

Shape into Bites:

1. Using clean hands, take small portions of the mixture and roll them into bite-sized balls. You can adjust the size to your preference.

2. Place the shaped protein bites on a parchment paper-lined tray or plate.

Chill and Set:

1. Place the tray of protein bites in the refrigerator for about 30 minutes. This helps them firm up and become easier to handle.

Store and Enjoy:

1. Once the protein bites have chilled and set, transfer them to an airtight container.

2. Store your Chocolate Protein Bites in the refrigerator for longer freshness.

Pro Tips:

- Customize your protein bites by adding ingredients like shredded coconut, chopped nuts, or dried fruits for extra texture and flavor.

- If the mixture is too dry, add a bit more honey or nut butter. If it's too sticky, add more oats or protein powder.

These Chocolate Protein Bites are a fantastic snack option for refueling after a workout or satisfying your chocolate cravings while supporting muscle growth and recovery. They are packed with protein and wholesome ingredients, making them a delicious and convenient choice.

5.7. Protein-Packed Rice Pudding

Ingredients:

- 1 cup cooked brown rice (preferably cooked in unsweetened almond milk)

- 2 cups unsweetened almond milk (or any milk of choice)

- 1/4 cup vanilla protein powder

- 2 tablespoons honey or maple syrup (adjust to your preferred level of sweetness)

- 1/2 teaspoon ground cinnamon

- 1/4 teaspoon vanilla extract

- A pinch of salt

- Chopped nuts or raisins for garnish (optional)

Instructions:

Prepare the Rice:

1. Cook the brown rice according to the package instructions, preferably using unsweetened almond milk instead of water. This adds creaminess and flavor to the rice.

Make the Pudding:

1. In a saucepan, combine the cooked brown rice, unsweetened almond milk, vanilla protein powder, honey or maple syrup, ground cinnamon, vanilla extract, and a pinch of salt.

2. Stir the mixture well to combine all the ingredients.

Simmer and Stir:

1. Place the saucepan over medium heat and bring the mixture to a gentle simmer. Stir frequently to prevent sticking or burning.

2. Let the pudding simmer for about 15-20 minutes, or until it thickens to your desired consistency. Keep in mind that it will thicken further as it cools.

Taste and Adjust:

1. Taste the protein-packed rice pudding and adjust the sweetness or cinnamon flavor to your liking. Add more honey, maple syrup, or cinnamon if desired.

Serve and Garnish:

1. Transfer the hot rice pudding to serving bowls.

2. Optionally, garnish with chopped nuts or raisins for added texture and flavor.

3. Serve your Protein-Packed Rice Pudding warm as a comforting and protein-rich dessert that's perfect for muscle recovery and satisfying your sweet tooth.

Pro Tips:

- Experiment with different milk alternatives like coconut milk or almond-coconut blend for unique flavors.

- Add a dash of nutmeg or a sprinkle of cocoa powder for extra flavor variety.

This Protein-Packed Rice Pudding is a delicious and nutritious dessert that combines the comfort of classic rice pudding with the benefits of added protein. It's a delightful way to treat yourself while supporting your muscle-building journey.

5.8. Almond and Date Protein Bars

Ingredients:

- 1 cup almonds

- 1 cup pitted Medjool dates (about 10-12 dates)

- 1/2 cup vanilla protein powder

- 1/4 cup unsweetened almond butter

- 1/4 cup unsweetened shredded coconut

- 1/4 cup water

- 1 teaspoon vanilla extract

- A pinch of salt

- Dark chocolate chips for drizzling (optional)

Instructions:

Prepare the Base:

1. In a food processor, add the almonds and pulse until they are finely ground into a coarse almond meal.

2. Add the pitted Medjool dates, vanilla protein powder, unsweetened almond butter, unsweetened shredded coconut, water, vanilla extract, and a pinch of salt to the almond meal in the food processor.

3. Process all the ingredients until the mixture comes together into a sticky dough-like consistency. You may need to stop and scrape down the sides of the food processor a few times to ensure thorough mixing.

Shape the Bars:

1. Line an 8x8-inch (20x20 cm) square baking pan with parchment paper, leaving some overhang on the sides for easy removal.

2. Transfer the mixture from the food processor into the lined baking pan.

3. Use clean hands or a spatula to press the mixture evenly into the pan, ensuring it's compact and smooth.

Chill and Set:

1. Place the pan in the refrigerator for about 30 minutes to allow the bars to firm up.

Cut and Drizzle (Optional):

1. Once the bars have set, use a sharp knife to cut them into your desired bar size or shape.

2. Optionally, melt some dark chocolate chips in the microwave or over a double boiler and drizzle the melted chocolate over the bars for added flavor and decoration.

Store and Enjoy:

1. Store your Almond and Date Protein Bars in an airtight container in the refrigerator for freshness.

2. Enjoy these protein-packed bars as a nutritious and satisfying dessert or snack that supports your muscle-building journey.

Pro Tips:

- Feel free to customize your protein bars with added ingredients like chia seeds, dried fruits, or your favorite nuts.

These Almond and Date Protein Bars are a delightful and convenient way to enjoy a protein-rich snack or dessert. They provide both the sweetness of dates and the crunch of almonds, making them a perfect choice for muscle recovery and a quick energy boost.

5.9. Chocolate Protein Pancakes

Ingredients:

- 1 cup rolled oats

- 2 tablespoons chocolate protein powder

- 2 ripe bananas

- 2 large eggs

- 1/4 cup unsweetened almond milk (or any milk of choice)

- 1 tablespoon unsweetened cocoa powder

- 1 teaspoon vanilla extract

- 1/2 teaspoon baking powder

- A pinch of salt

- Cooking spray or a bit of coconut oil for the pan

Instructions:

Prepare the Pancake Batter:

1. In a blender, combine the rolled oats, chocolate protein powder, ripe bananas, large eggs, unsweetened almond milk, unsweetened cocoa powder, vanilla extract, baking powder, and a pinch of salt.

2. Blend all the ingredients until you have a smooth pancake batter. Make sure there are no lumps.

Heat the Pan:

1. Heat a non-stick skillet or griddle over medium heat and lightly grease it with cooking spray or a bit of coconut oil.

Cook the Pancakes:

1. Pour small ladlefuls of the pancake batter onto the hot skillet, creating pancakes of your desired size. You can adjust the size based on your preference.

2. Cook the pancakes for about 2-3 minutes on each side or until they are golden brown and slightly puffed. Bubbles may form on the surface as a sign that it's time to flip them.

Serve and Enjoy:

1. Once the pancakes are cooked to perfection, transfer them to a serving plate.

2. Optionally, garnish with fresh berries, a dollop of Greek yogurt, or a drizzle of maple syrup for extra flavor.

3. Serve your Chocolate Protein Pancakes immediately as a delightful and protein-rich breakfast or dessert option that supports your muscle-building journey.

Pro Tips:

- Customize your pancakes by adding chocolate chips, chopped nuts, or sliced bananas to the batter before cooking.

- Experiment with different flavors of protein powder for variety.

These Chocolate Protein Pancakes are a scrumptious and nutritious twist on traditional

5.10. Protein-Rich Chia Pudding

Ingredients:

- 1/4 cup chia seeds

- 1 cup unsweetened almond milk (or any milk of choice)

- 1/4 cup vanilla protein powder

- 1 tablespoon honey or maple syrup (adjust to your preferred level of sweetness)

- 1/2 teaspoon vanilla extract

- A pinch of salt

- Fresh berries or sliced fruit for topping (optional)

- Chopped nuts or shredded coconut for garnish (optional)

Instructions:

Prepare the Pudding Base:

1. In a mixing bowl, combine the chia seeds, unsweetened almond milk, vanilla protein powder, honey or maple syrup, vanilla extract, and a pinch of salt.

2. Stir the mixture well to ensure the chia seeds are evenly distributed and not clumped together.

Chill and Set:

1. Cover the bowl and refrigerate the protein-rich chia pudding mixture for at least 4 hours or overnight. This allows the chia seeds to absorb the liquid and create a pudding-like texture. Stir it once or twice during this time to prevent clumping.

Serve and Garnish:

1. When ready to serve, give the chia pudding a good stir to make sure it's well combined.

2. Optionally, top your Protein-Rich Chia Pudding with fresh berries or sliced fruit for natural sweetness and a pop of color.

3. Garnish with chopped nuts or shredded coconut for added texture and flavor.

4. Serve your chia pudding as a protein-packed and satisfying dessert or breakfast option that aligns perfectly with your muscle-building journey.

Pro Tips:

- Experiment with different flavors of protein powder to create unique variations of chia pudding.

- Add a sprinkle of cinnamon or a drizzle of nut butter for extra flavor complexity.

This Protein-Rich Chia Pudding is a convenient and wholesome dessert or breakfast choice that's rich in protein and essential nutrients. It's a delightful way to treat yourself while nourishing your muscles.

CHAPTER 6: SIDES AND EXTRAS

In this chapter, we'll explore a variety of side dishes and extras that complement your main meals. These additions not only enhance the flavor of your dishes but also provide additional nutrients to support your muscle-building journey. From nutrient-packed salads to savory accompaniments, these recipes will take your meals to the next level.

6.1. Quinoa and Black Bean Salad

Ingredients:

For the Salad:

- 1 cup quinoa, rinsed and cooked according to package instructions

- 1 can (15 ounces) black beans, drained and rinsed

- 1 cup corn kernels (fresh, frozen, or canned)

- 1 red bell pepper, diced

- 1/2 cup diced red onion

- 1/4 cup chopped fresh cilantro or parsley

For the Dressing:

- 1/4 cup olive oil

- 2 tablespoons fresh lime juice

- 1 clove garlic, minced

- 1 teaspoon ground cumin

- 1/2 teaspoon chili powder

- Salt and black pepper to taste

Instructions:

Prepare the Salad:

1. Cook the quinoa according to the package instructions. Once cooked, let it cool to room temperature.

2. In a large mixing bowl, combine the cooked quinoa, black beans, corn kernels, diced red bell pepper, diced red onion, and chopped cilantro or parsley.

Make the Dressing:

1. In a separate small bowl, whisk together the olive oil, fresh lime juice, minced garlic, ground cumin, chili powder, salt, and black pepper. Mix until the dressing is well combined.

Combine and Toss:

1. Pour the dressing over the quinoa and black bean salad.

2. Gently toss all the ingredients together until the salad is evenly coated with the dressing.

Chill and Serve:

1. Cover the salad bowl and refrigerate for at least 30 minutes before serving. This allows the flavors to meld and the salad to chill.

2. Serve your Quinoa and Black Bean Salad as a flavorful and protein-rich side dish or add grilled chicken or tofu to turn it into a satisfying main meal that supports your muscle-building goals.

Pro Tips:

- Customize the salad by adding diced avocado, cherry tomatoes, or jalapeños for extra flavor and variety.

- This salad can be made ahead and stored in the refrigerator for a day or two, making it a convenient option for meal prep.

This Quinoa and Black Bean Salad is a nutritious and satisfying side dish that's packed with protein, fiber, and essential nutrients. It's a flavorful addition to your meals that complements your muscle-building journey.

6.2. Garlic Roasted Broccoli

Ingredients:

- 1 pound (about 450 grams) fresh broccoli florets

- 3 cloves garlic, minced

- 2 tablespoons olive oil

- 1/2 teaspoon salt

- 1/4 teaspoon black pepper

- 1/4 teaspoon red pepper flakes (optional, for a bit of heat)

- Zest of 1 lemon (optional, for a burst of freshness)

- Grated Parmesan cheese for garnish (optional)

Instructions:

Prepare the Broccoli:

1. Preheat your oven to 425°F (220°C). Line a baking sheet with parchment paper or lightly grease it.

2. Wash and thoroughly dry the broccoli florets. Make sure they are completely dry to achieve a crispy texture when roasted.

Season the Broccoli:

1. In a large mixing bowl, combine the dry broccoli florets, minced garlic, olive oil, salt, black pepper, and red pepper flakes (if using). Toss everything together until the broccoli is evenly coated with the seasonings.

Roast the Broccoli:

1. Spread the seasoned broccoli florets in a single layer on the prepared baking sheet.

2. Roast in the preheated oven for 20-25 minutes or until the broccoli is tender and slightly crispy at the edges. Be sure to give it a gentle toss or shake the pan halfway through the roasting time for even cooking.

Garnish and Serve:

1. Once the garlic roasted broccoli is done, remove it from the oven.

2. Optionally, garnish with lemon zest for a burst of freshness and grated Parmesan cheese for extra flavor.

3. Serve your Garlic Roasted Broccoli as a delicious and nutritious side dish that pairs perfectly with your main meals while supporting your muscle-building journey.

Pro Tips:

- Customize your roasted broccoli by adding a squeeze of lemon juice or a sprinkle of your favorite herbs and spices.

- To make it a complete meal, toss in some roasted chickpeas or grilled chicken before serving.

This Garlic Roasted Broccoli is a flavorful and wholesome side dish that's rich in vitamins, minerals, and fiber. It's a fantastic addition to your meals, providing both taste and nutrition.

6.3. Sweet Potato Fries

Ingredients:

- 2 large sweet potatoes, peeled and cut into matchstick fries

- 2 tablespoons olive oil

- 1 teaspoon paprika

- 1/2 teaspoon garlic powder

- 1/2 teaspoon onion powder

- 1/2 teaspoon salt

- 1/4 teaspoon black pepper

- Fresh parsley or cilantro for garnish (optional)

- Dipping sauce of your choice (such as yogurt-based or ketchup)

Instructions:

Prepare the Sweet Potatoes:

1. Preheat your oven to 425°F (220°C). Line a baking sheet with parchment paper or lightly grease it.

2. Peel the sweet potatoes and cut them into matchstick-sized fries. Make sure they are of uniform size for even cooking.

Season the Fries:

1. In a large mixing bowl, combine the sweet potato fries, olive oil, paprika, garlic powder, onion powder, salt, and black pepper. Toss everything together until the fries are evenly coated with the seasonings.

Bake the Fries:

1. Spread the seasoned sweet potato fries in a single layer on the prepared baking sheet, ensuring they are not overcrowded.

2. Bake in the preheated oven for 25-30 minutes, flipping the fries halfway through, or until they are crispy and golden brown.

Garnish and Serve:

1. Once the sweet potato fries are done, remove them from the oven.

2. Optionally, garnish with fresh parsley or cilantro for added freshness.

3. Serve your Sweet Potato Fries hot with a dipping sauce of your choice. They make a tasty and nutritious side dish that complements your muscle-building meals.

Pro Tips:

- Experiment with different seasonings like rosemary, thyme, or smoked paprika for unique flavor variations.

- For a crispier texture, make sure the fries are spread out in a single layer on the baking sheet without overcrowding.

These Sweet Potato Fries are a flavorful and nutritious alternative to traditional fries. They are rich in vitamins, fiber, and complex carbohydrates, making them a perfect side dish to fuel your muscles.

6.4. Spinach and Feta Stuffed Mushrooms

Ingredients:

- 12 large white mushrooms, cleaned and stems removed

- 2 cups fresh spinach, chopped

- 1/2 cup crumbled feta cheese

- 2 cloves garlic, minced

- 2 tablespoons olive oil

- Salt and black pepper to taste

- Fresh parsley for garnish (optional)

Instructions:

Prepare the Mushrooms:

1. Preheat your oven to 375°F (190°C). Line a baking sheet with parchment paper.

2. Clean the mushrooms with a damp paper towel to remove any dirt. Gently remove the stems, creating a hollow space for the stuffing. Set the mushroom caps aside.

Prepare the Filling:

1. In a skillet, heat the olive oil over medium heat. Add the minced garlic and sauté for about 1 minute until fragrant.

2. Add the chopped spinach to the skillet and sauté for 2-3 minutes until it wilts. Season with a pinch of salt and black pepper.

3. Remove the skillet from heat and stir in the crumbled feta cheese. Mix until the cheese is evenly distributed in the spinach mixture.

Stuff the Mushrooms:

1. Take each mushroom cap and stuff it generously with the spinach and feta filling. Press the filling gently to pack it into the mushrooms.

2. Place the stuffed mushrooms on the prepared baking sheet.

Bake:

1. Bake the stuffed mushrooms in the preheated oven for about 15-20 minutes or until the mushrooms are tender and the filling is slightly golden on top.

Garnish and Serve:

1. Once done, remove the stuffed mushrooms from the oven.

2. Optionally, garnish with fresh parsley for added color and flavor.

3. Serve your Spinach and Feta Stuffed Mushrooms as a delectable and protein-rich side dish or appetizer that adds a burst of taste to your muscle-building meals.

Pro Tips:

- Experiment with different cheese options like goat cheese or mozzarella for varied flavors.

- You can also sprinkle some breadcrumbs on top of the filling for a crispy texture.

These Spinach and Feta Stuffed Mushrooms are a delightful and nutritious addition to your meal. Packed with protein and wholesome ingredients, they are a flavorful way to support your muscle-building journey.

6.5. Grilled Asparagus with Lemon

Ingredients:

- 1 bunch of fresh asparagus spears, woody ends trimmed

- 2 tablespoons olive oil

- Zest of 1 lemon

- Juice of 1 lemon

- 2 cloves garlic, minced

- Salt and black pepper to taste

- Fresh parsley or grated Parmesan cheese for garnish (optional)

Instructions:

Prepare the Asparagus:

1. Preheat your grill to medium-high heat.

2. Trim the woody ends of the asparagus spears to ensure they are tender and delicious.

Marinate the Asparagus:

1. In a bowl, combine the olive oil, lemon zest, lemon juice, minced garlic, salt, and black pepper. Mix well to create a marinade.

2. Place the trimmed asparagus spears in a shallow dish and pour the marinade over them. Toss the asparagus to ensure they are evenly coated with the marinade. Let them sit for about 10 minutes to soak in the flavors.

Grill the Asparagus:

1. Place the marinated asparagus spears directly on the preheated grill.

2. Grill for approximately 5-7 minutes, turning occasionally, until the asparagus is tender and has grill marks.

Garnish and Serve:

1. Once done, remove the grilled asparagus from the grill.

2. Optionally, garnish with fresh parsley or grated Parmesan cheese for added freshness and flavor.

3. Serve your Grilled Asparagus with Lemon as a delightful and nutrient-rich side dish that complements your muscle-building meals.

Pro Tips:

- If you don't have a grill, you can achieve similar results by roasting the marinated asparagus in a preheated oven at 425°F (220°C) for about 15-20 minutes.

This Grilled Asparagus with Lemon is a simple yet flavorful side dish that adds a burst of freshness to your meal. It's packed with vitamins and minerals, making it a fantastic choice for supporting your muscle-building journey.

CHAPTER 7: EXPERT ADVICE AND TIPS

In this chapter, we provide you with valuable insights and expert advice to help you make the most out of your muscle-building journey. Building and maintaining muscle requires more than just nutritious recipes; it involves a comprehensive understanding of fitness, nutrition, and lifestyle. Here, you'll find tips, tricks, and guidance from fitness and nutrition experts to support your goals.

7.1. Nutrient Timing for Muscle Growth

Achieving your muscle-building goals isn't just about what you eat but also when you eat. Nutrient timing plays a vital role in maximizing muscle growth and recovery. In this section, we'll delve into the science and strategies behind nutrient timing for muscle development.

Understanding the Anabolic Window

The concept of an "anabolic window" refers to the period following your workout when your muscles are primed for nutrient uptake and growth. This window typically lasts for about 30 minutes to 2 hours post-exercise, although it's not as rigid as once believed. During this time, your body is more receptive to nutrients, especially protein, carbohydrates, and certain vitamins and minerals.

Protein Power Post-Workout

Protein is a cornerstone of muscle growth, and post-workout is a crucial time to consume it. Here's why:

- **Muscle Protein Synthesis (MPS):** After exercise, your body undergoes a process called Muscle Protein Synthesis, where it repairs and builds muscle tissue. Protein provides the amino acids necessary for this process.

- **Recovery:** Protein intake post-workout helps reduce muscle soreness and accelerates recovery. It repairs micro-tears in muscle fibers caused by exercise.

- **Leucine's Role:** Leucine, an amino acid found in protein, plays a significant role in stimulating MPS. Aim for protein sources rich in leucine, such as lean meats, dairy, and plant-based options like soy and quinoa.

Carbohydrates Count

Carbohydrates are often overlooked post-workout, but they play a vital role:

- **Restoring Glycogen:** Intense exercise depletes glycogen stores in your muscles and liver. Consuming carbs post-workout replenishes these stores, ensuring you have the energy for your next workout.

- **Enhancing Protein Uptake:** Carbs stimulate the release of insulin, which helps drive amino acids from protein into your muscle cells. This enhances muscle protein synthesis.

Fats and Fiber

While protein and carbs take center stage post-workout, don't forget about healthy fats and fiber:

- **Healthy Fats:** Include sources like avocados, nuts, and olive oil in your post-workout meals. Fats aid in the absorption of fat-soluble vitamins and provide lasting energy.

- **Fiber:** Fiber aids digestion and helps stabilize blood sugar levels. While you don't need a lot of fiber immediately after a workout, consider adding some to your post-workout meal for overall health.

Hydration Matters

Proper hydration is essential for muscle function and recovery. Dehydration can lead to decreased performance and hinder muscle growth. Remember to drink water before, during, and after your workout to stay adequately hydrated.

Balanced Meals Post-Workout

Incorporating these principles into your post-workout meals can optimize muscle growth:

- **Protein and Carbs:** Consume a balanced meal that includes protein and carbohydrates within 30 minutes to 2 hours post-exercise.

- **Snacks or Shakes:** If you can't have a full meal immediately, opt for a protein shake or a snack that combines protein and carbs for quick recovery.

Tailoring to Your Needs

Remember that nutrient timing can vary based on individual factors like workout intensity, goals, and dietary preferences. The key is consistency. Ensure you consistently refuel your body post-workout with the nutrients it needs to recover and grow.

By understanding nutrient timing, you'll harness the power of your body's natural processes to support muscle growth effectively. The recipes in this cookbook are designed to help you meet your nutrient needs at the right times, so you can fuel your workouts and achieve your muscle-building goals.

7.2. Grocery Shopping for Muscle Builders

Building and maintaining muscle requires a well-planned diet that provides the necessary nutrients for growth and recovery. To set yourself up for success, it all starts with smart grocery shopping. In this section, we'll guide you through the aisles to help you make the right choices for your muscle-building journey.

Create a Shopping List

Before heading to the store, create a shopping list based on your meal plan and the recipes in this cookbook. Having a list ensures you purchase everything you need and reduces the temptation to buy unnecessary items.

Prioritize Lean Proteins

Protein is the building block of muscle, so it's essential to include lean protein sources in your shopping list:

- **Poultry:** Skinless chicken breast and turkey.

- **Lean Meats:** Beef cuts like sirloin or tenderloin, and pork loin.

- **Fish:** Salmon, tuna, cod, and other varieties rich in omega-3 fatty acids.

- **Plant-Based Proteins:** Tofu, tempeh, legumes (beans, lentils, chickpeas), and quinoa.

Choose Complex Carbohydrates

Carbohydrates provide the energy needed for intense workouts and muscle recovery. Opt for complex carbs that offer sustained energy:

- **Whole Grains:** Brown rice, quinoa, whole wheat pasta, and oats.

- **Starchy Vegetables:** Sweet potatoes, regular potatoes, and corn.

- **Fruits:** Berries, apples, bananas, and citrus fruits.

Don't Forget Healthy Fats

Healthy fats are crucial for overall health and hormone production, which impacts muscle growth:

- **Avocado**

- **Nuts and Seeds:** Almonds, walnuts, chia seeds, and flaxseeds.

- **Olive Oil and Coconut Oil**

Load Up on Veggies

Vegetables are rich in vitamins, minerals, and antioxidants that support muscle health and recovery:

- **Leafy Greens:** Spinach, kale, and Swiss chard.

- **Colorful Veggies:** Bell peppers, carrots, and broccoli.

- **Cruciferous Veggies:** Cauliflower, Brussels sprouts, and cabbage.

Dairy and Dairy Alternatives

Dairy and dairy alternatives are excellent sources of calcium and protein:

- **Greek Yogurt:** High in protein and probiotics.

- **Milk:** Cow's milk or plant-based options like almond or soy milk.

- **Cheese:** Choose low-fat or reduced-fat varieties.

Plan for Snacks and Supplements

- Stock up on healthy snacks like mixed nuts, Greek yogurt, and protein bars for quick refueling.

- Consider your supplement needs, such as protein powder, creatine, or branched-chain amino acids (BCAAs).

Read Labels

When selecting packaged foods, read labels to check for added sugars, excessive sodium, and artificial additives. Look for whole, minimally processed options whenever possible.

Shop the Perimeter

In most grocery stores, the perimeter is where you'll find fresh produce, lean meats, and dairy products. Focus on these sections for the majority of your shopping to avoid highly processed foods in the center aisles.

Meal Prep Essentials

Invest in containers and storage solutions for meal prep. Having a well-organized kitchen makes it easier to prepare and store your muscle-building meals.

Stay Hydrated

Don't forget to include water on your shopping list. Proper hydration is crucial for muscle function and recovery.

Plan Ahead and Stay Consistent

Effective grocery shopping is all about planning and consistency. Stick to your list, avoid impulse purchases, and make grocery shopping a regular part of your routine to support your muscle-building goals.

With the right foods in your kitchen, you'll be well-prepared to follow the recipes in this cookbook and make smart nutritional choices to fuel your muscles effectively.

7.3. Portion Control and Meal Planning

Achieving your muscle-building goals requires more than just eating the right foods; it involves understanding portion control and planning your meals strategically. In this section, we'll explore the importance of portion sizes and how to create balanced meals that support muscle growth.

The Role of Portion Control

Portion control is the practice of managing the quantity of food you consume in a single serving. It plays a vital role in both muscle building and maintaining a healthy weight. Here's why it matters:

Preventing Overconsumption: Eating too much, even of healthy foods, can lead to excess calorie intake, which may result in unwanted weight gain.

Optimizing Nutrient Intake: Proper portion control ensures you get the right balance of macronutrients (protein, carbohydrates, and fats) and essential vitamins and minerals in each meal.

Avoiding Energy Dips: Overeating can lead to energy crashes and sluggishness, which can impact your workout performance and daily activities.

Balanced Meals for Muscle Growth

To support your muscle-building journey, aim for balanced meals that incorporate the following elements:

Protein: Include a lean source of protein in each meal. Protein is crucial for muscle repair and growth. Good options include lean meats, poultry, fish, tofu, legumes, and dairy products.

Carbohydrates: Incorporate complex carbohydrates to provide sustained energy for workouts and recovery. Whole grains, starchy vegetables, and fruits are excellent choices.

Healthy Fats: Include healthy fats from sources like avocados, nuts, and olive oil. Fats aid in the absorption of fat-soluble vitamins and provide essential nutrients.

Fiber: Fiber-rich foods like vegetables, whole grains, and legumes help with digestion, keep you feeling full, and stabilize blood sugar levels.

Hydration: Don't forget to drink water throughout the day to stay well-hydrated. Proper hydration is essential for muscle function and overall health.

Meal Planning Tips

Effective meal planning simplifies the process of creating balanced meals and ensures you have the right foods on hand. Here are some tips:

Plan Ahead: Take time each week to plan your meals and snacks. Consider using a meal planning app or calendar to keep track.

Batch Cooking: Prepare larger quantities of certain dishes and freeze them in individual portions. This makes it easy to grab a balanced meal when you're short on time.

Protein Priority: Plan your meals around your protein source, then add vegetables and carbs. For example, if you choose grilled chicken as your protein, build the meal with vegetables and a whole grain like quinoa.

Snack Smart: Plan for healthy snacks between meals to maintain energy levels and support muscle recovery. Opt for options like Greek yogurt, mixed nuts, or protein-rich smoothies.

Flexible Options: Keep some versatile ingredients on hand that can be used in various recipes, like canned beans, frozen vegetables, and brown rice.

Stay Consistent: Try to eat at regular intervals to maintain steady energy levels and support your workouts.

By practicing portion control and thoughtful meal planning, you'll ensure that your diet is optimized for muscle growth while avoiding overconsumption. The recipes in this cookbook are designed to help you create balanced and delicious meals that support your fitness goals.

7.4. Adapting Recipes to Dietary Preferences

Eating for muscle building doesn't mean you have to follow a one-size-fits-all approach. Everyone's dietary preferences and needs vary. In this section, we'll explore how to adapt the recipes in this cookbook to accommodate different dietary preferences, including vegetarian, vegan, gluten-free, and more.

Vegetarian and Vegan Options

For those who prefer plant-based diets, you can easily adapt recipes to be vegetarian or vegan:

- **Protein Sources:** Substitute animal-based proteins with plant-based options like tofu, tempeh, seitan, legumes (beans, lentils, chickpeas), and plant-based protein sources (such as pea or soy protein).

- **Dairy Alternatives:** Replace dairy products with plant-based alternatives like almond milk, soy yogurt, and vegan cheese.

- **Egg Replacements:** In baking or breakfast recipes that call for eggs, use egg replacers like flaxseed meal, chia seeds, or commercial egg substitutes.

Gluten-Free Choices

If you follow a gluten-free diet due to celiac disease or gluten sensitivity, you can still enjoy muscle-building meals:

- **Grains:** Substitute wheat-based grains with gluten-free alternatives like quinoa, rice, gluten-free oats, and corn-based products.

- **Flour Alternatives:** In baking recipes, use gluten-free flours like almond flour, coconut flour, or a gluten-free flour blend.

- **Gluten-Free Products:** Look for gluten-free versions of pasta, bread, and other staples when needed.

Low-Carb and Keto-Friendly Modifications

If you're following a low-carb or keto diet to support your muscle-building goals, consider the following adaptations:

- **Carb Reduction:** Decrease the amount of high-carb ingredients like grains and starchy vegetables in recipes.

- **Increase Healthy Fats:** Incorporate more healthy fats like avocado, olive oil, nuts, and seeds into your meals.

- **Sugar Alternatives:** Use sugar substitutes like stevia, erythritol, or monk fruit sweetener in dessert recipes.

Allergen-Free Alternatives

If you have allergies or dietary restrictions, there are ways to adapt recipes to accommodate your needs:

- **Nut Allergies:** Choose recipes that are nut-free and use seeds or seed butter instead.

- **Dairy Allergies:** Opt for dairy-free alternatives like almond milk, coconut yogurt, or vegan cheese.

- **Soy Allergies:** Swap out soy-based products for alternatives like almond tofu or chickpea-based options.

Customizing Flavor Profiles

Feel free to experiment with herbs, spices, and seasonings to customize the flavors of your dishes. Different combinations can make the same base recipe taste entirely different.

Portion Control and Macronutrient Balancing

Regardless of your dietary preferences, you can still practice portion control and balance your macronutrients (protein, carbs, fats) to meet your muscle-building goals.

By adapting the recipes in this cookbook to your specific dietary preferences, you'll be able to enjoy delicious and nutritious meals that align with your individual needs and support your muscle-building journey.

7.5. Staying Committed to Your Muscle-Building Journey

Building and maintaining muscle requires dedication and commitment. Staying on track with your goals involves more than just following recipes; it's about adopting a sustainable and focused lifestyle. In this section, we'll explore strategies to help you stay committed to your muscle-building journey.

Set Realistic Goals

Begin by setting clear, achievable goals. Whether you're aiming to gain muscle, lose fat, or improve your overall fitness, having well-defined objectives provides motivation and direction.

Track Your Progress

Monitoring your progress is essential for staying committed. Keep a workout journal to record your exercises, weights, and repetitions. Take measurements and photos regularly to visually track your changes.

Stay Consistent

Consistency is key to success. Stick to your workout routine and meal plan. Avoid skipping workouts or indulging in unhealthy foods too frequently. Consistency builds habits that lead to lasting results.

Find a Support System

Having a support system can be invaluable. Share your goals with friends or family who can encourage and motivate you. Consider joining a fitness community or finding a workout partner who shares your objectives.

Plan and Prepare

Prepare your meals in advance to avoid impulsive, unhealthy choices. Having nutritious meals readily available makes it easier to stay on track. Use the recipes in this cookbook for convenient and balanced options.

Listen to Your Body

Pay attention to your body's signals. Rest when needed, and don't push through pain or fatigue that may lead to injury. Adequate rest and recovery are crucial for muscle growth.

Stay Educated

Continue learning about fitness and nutrition. Stay updated on the latest research and trends in muscle building. Knowledge empowers you to make informed choices.

Adapt to Challenges

Expect challenges and setbacks along the way. Life can be unpredictable, but adaptability is a valuable skill. If you miss a workout or have an off day, don't be discouraged. Get back on track as soon as possible.

Celebrate Achievements

Acknowledge your accomplishments, no matter how small. Celebrate reaching milestones and achieving your goals. Rewarding yourself reinforces positive behaviors.

Mindset Matters

Maintain a positive mindset. Visualize your success and stay optimistic, even during tough times. A strong mental attitude can help you overcome obstacles.

Stay Hydrated and Rested

Proper hydration and quality sleep are essential for muscle recovery and overall health. Prioritize these aspects of your well-being to support your journey.

Remember Why You Started

When faced with challenges or moments of doubt, reflect on why you started this journey. Your initial motivation can reignite your commitment.

Seek Professional Guidance

Consider working with a fitness trainer or a nutritionist. They can provide personalized guidance, tailor your plan to your specific needs, and offer expert advice.

Stay Inspired

Find inspiration from role models in the fitness industry or individuals who have achieved similar goals. Their success stories can serve as motivation.

Building muscle is a journey that requires dedication and perseverance. By implementing these strategies and staying committed to your goals, you'll be well-equipped to succeed in your muscle-building journey.

7.6. Pre- and Post-Workout Nutrition

Optimizing your nutrition before and after your workouts is essential for maximizing muscle growth and recovery. In this section, we'll explore the science behind pre- and post-workout nutrition and provide expert tips on fueling your body effectively.

7.6.1: Pre-Workout Nutrition

Before you hit the gym, it's crucial to provide your body with the right nutrients for energy and performance. Here's how to prepare your pre-workout meal:

Timing Matters: Aim to eat a balanced meal or snack 1-3 hours before your workout. This allows your body to digest and absorb the nutrients.

Carbohydrates for Energy: Consume complex carbohydrates like whole grains, fruits, or starchy vegetables. Carbs provide a readily available energy source for your muscles.

Protein for Muscle Support: Include a moderate amount of protein to prevent muscle breakdown. Lean protein sources like chicken, turkey, tofu, or Greek yogurt are excellent choices.

Hydration: Hydrate adequately before your workout. Dehydration can lead to decreased performance and muscle cramps.

7.6.2: Post-Workout Nutrition

After an intense workout, your body is primed for nutrient absorption and muscle repair. Here's how to make the most of your post-workout meal:

Protein for Recovery: Within 30 minutes to 2 hours post-exercise, consume a meal or snack rich in protein. This supports muscle protein synthesis and recovery.

Carbohydrates for Glycogen Replenishment: Include carbohydrates to replenish glycogen stores in your muscles. This helps with recovery and energy for your next workout.

Lean Protein Sources: Opt for lean proteins like chicken, fish, beans, or plant-based options to reduce fat intake.

Healthy Fats: Incorporate healthy fats to aid in nutrient absorption and overall health. Avocado, nuts, and olive oil are great choices.

Hydration: Rehydrate with water or a balanced electrolyte drink to replace fluids lost during your workout.

Balanced Meals: Post-workout meals should be balanced with a mix of macronutrients (protein, carbs, fats) and include vegetables or fruits for vitamins and minerals.

Supplements: Consider adding a post-workout protein shake or supplement to ensure you're meeting your protein needs.

7.6.3: Snacking for Quick Recovery

If you have limited time between your workout and your next meal, opt for a quick and balanced snack that combines protein and carbohydrates. Protein bars, Greek yogurt with berries, or a smoothie with protein powder are convenient choices.

7.6.4: Personalizing Your Pre- and Post-Workout Nutrition

Remember that individual preferences and needs vary. Experiment with different foods and timing to discover what works best for your body. Pay attention to how you feel during and after workouts to make adjustments.

7.6.5: Hydration for Optimal Performance

Proper hydration is essential for muscle function and overall performance. Drink water before, during, and after your workouts. Consider electrolyte drinks for intense or prolonged exercise.

By paying attention to your pre- and post-workout nutrition, you'll provide your body with the fuel it needs to perform at its best and recover effectively. The recipes in this cookbook are designed to support your muscle-building goals by offering nutritious options for both pre- and post-workout meals.

7.7. Supplements for Muscle Support

While a well-balanced diet should provide most of the nutrients you need for muscle building, there are specific supplements that can complement your nutrition plan and support your muscle-building goals. In this section, we'll explore common supplements used by individuals focused on muscle support.

7.7.1: Protein Supplements

Whey Protein: Whey protein is a fast-digesting protein source commonly used for muscle recovery. It's rich in essential amino acids and is quickly absorbed, making it an excellent choice for post-workout shakes.

Casein Protein: Casein protein is slower-digesting and provides a steady release of amino acids into the bloodstream. It's often consumed before bedtime to support overnight muscle recovery.

Plant-Based Protein: For those following a vegetarian or vegan diet, plant-based protein powders like pea, soy, or rice protein can be excellent options to meet protein needs.

7.7.2: Creatine

Creatine is a well-researched supplement that can enhance muscle strength and power. It works by increasing the body's production of adenosine triphosphate (ATP), which fuels muscle contractions. Creatine is commonly taken as a daily supplement, with a typical dosage of 3-5 grams per day.

7.7.3: Branched-Chain Amino Acids (BCAAs)

BCAAs, including leucine, isoleucine, and valine, are essential amino acids that play a role in muscle protein synthesis. They are often used to support muscle recovery and reduce muscle soreness. BCAA supplements can be taken before, during, or after workouts.

7.7.4: Beta-Alanine

Beta-alanine is an amino acid that combines with histidine to form carnosine in the muscles. Carnosine helps buffer the build-up of lactic acid during exercise, reducing muscle fatigue and improving endurance. A common dosage is 3-6 grams per day.

7.7.5: Glutamine

Glutamine is an amino acid that plays a role in muscle recovery and immune system support. While it can be obtained through dietary sources, some individuals choose to supplement with glutamine to aid in muscle repair. Typical dosages range from 5-10 grams per day.

7.7.6: Multivitamins and Minerals

A high-quality multivitamin and mineral supplement can ensure you're meeting your micronutrient needs, especially if your diet is restricted or lacks variety. Look for a supplement that includes essential vitamins and minerals like vitamin D, calcium, magnesium, and zinc.

7.7.7: Omega-3 Fatty Acids

Omega-3 fatty acids, commonly found in fish oil supplements, offer anti-inflammatory benefits and support overall health. While not directly related to muscle building, reducing inflammation can aid in recovery and joint health.

7.7.8: Pre-Workout Supplements

Pre-workout supplements often contain a combination of ingredients like caffeine, beta-alanine, and nitric oxide boosters. They can provide a temporary energy boost and enhance workout performance. Use these supplements with caution and follow recommended dosages.

7.7.9: Consultation with a Healthcare Professional

Before adding supplements to your routine, consider consulting with a healthcare professional or a registered dietitian. They can assess your individual needs and provide personalized recommendations based on your goals, dietary habits, and any potential health concerns.

Supplements should complement a well-rounded diet and should not be used as a substitute for whole foods. It's important to prioritize nutritious meals and use supplements when necessary to fill specific nutritional gaps or enhance performance.

7.8. Rest and Recovery

Rest and recovery are integral parts of any effective muscle-building program. While nutrition and exercise are essential, giving your body time to recuperate is equally crucial. In this section, we'll explore the importance of rest and recovery and provide tips on how to optimize this vital aspect of your muscle-building journey.

7.8.1: The Role of Rest in Muscle Building

Muscles grow and repair during periods of rest, not just during workouts. Here's why rest is essential:

Muscle Repair: During workouts, tiny muscle fibers experience micro-tears. Rest allows these fibers to repair and grow stronger.

Hormone Production: Adequate rest supports hormone production, including testosterone and growth hormone, both crucial for muscle growth.

Central Nervous System Recovery: Intense workouts stress the central nervous system. Rest helps it recover, leading to better performance in subsequent workouts.

Section 7.8.2: Quality Sleep for Recovery

Quality sleep is a cornerstone of recovery. Aim for 7-9 hours of uninterrupted sleep per night. Here's why sleep matters:

Muscle Growth: Growth hormone is released during deep sleep phases, promoting muscle recovery and repair.

Energy Restoration: Sleep restores glycogen levels, providing energy for your workouts.

Cognitive Function: Sleep is crucial for mental clarity, focus, and mood, all of which impact your motivation and performance.

7.8.3: Active Recovery

Active recovery involves low-intensity activities that promote blood flow without causing muscle fatigue. Activities like walking, cycling, or yoga can aid recovery by:

Reducing Muscle Soreness: Light movement can alleviate muscle stiffness and soreness.

Enhancing Circulation: Active recovery helps transport nutrients and oxygen to muscles, aiding in repair.

Mental Relaxation: It can serve as a mental break from intense training, reducing stress.

7.8.4: Nutrition for Recovery

Nutrition plays a vital role in recovery. Ensure your post-workout meals contain a balance of protein, carbohydrates, and healthy fats to support muscle repair and replenish energy stores.

7.8.5: Hydration for Recovery

Proper hydration is essential for muscle function and recovery. Drink water regularly to avoid dehydration, which can hinder recovery.

7.8.6: Listening to Your Body

Pay attention to your body's signals. If you're feeling fatigued or experiencing pain beyond typical muscle soreness, it may be a sign that you need more rest.

7.8.7: Active Recovery Days

Incorporate active recovery days into your weekly routine. These days can involve lighter workouts or activities like stretching, mobility work, or swimming.

7.8.8: Rest Days

Scheduled rest days are crucial. Plan these days to allow your muscles and central nervous system to recover fully. Use the time to relax, catch up on sleep, and recharge.

7.8.9: Reducing Stress

Stress, both physical and mental, can hinder recovery. Incorporate stress-reduction techniques like meditation, deep breathing, or hobbies you enjoy.

7.8.10: Consistency is Key

Consistently prioritize rest and recovery as part of your overall fitness routine. Over time, this dedication will contribute to your progress and overall well-being.

Remember that recovery is a personal journey, and what works best for one person may differ for another. Listen to your body, adjust your routine as needed, and make rest and recovery integral components of your muscle-building strategy.

7.9. Setting and Adjusting Goals

Setting clear and achievable goals is essential for success in your muscle-building journey. In this section, we'll explore the importance of goal setting, how to establish meaningful objectives, and the process of adjusting your goals as you progress.

7.9.1: The Power of Goal Setting

Setting specific goals provides direction, motivation, and a sense of purpose. Here's why goal setting matters:

Motivation: Clear goals give you something to strive for, keeping you motivated and focused.

Measuring Progress: Goals provide a way to measure your progress and track your achievements.

Accountability: Goals hold you accountable for your actions and help you stay committed.

7.9.2: SMART Goals

To ensure your goals are effective, follow the SMART criteria:

- **Specific:** Clearly define your goal. Instead of "I want to build muscle," specify, "I want to gain 10 pounds of lean muscle mass."

- **Measurable:** Set goals that you can track, like lifting a certain weight or reaching a specific body fat percentage.

- **Achievable:** Make sure your goals are realistic and attainable within your current circumstances.

- **Relevant:** Ensure your goals align with your overall muscle-building aspirations.

- **Time-Bound:** Set a deadline for achieving your goal, creating a sense of urgency.

7.9.3: Short-Term and Long-Term Goals

Create both short-term and long-term goals:

- **Short-Term Goals:** These are achievable in the near future, such as increasing your bench press by 10 pounds in the next three months.

- **Long-Term Goals:** These are larger, overarching objectives that may take several months or even years to achieve, such as transforming your overall physique.

7.9.4: Monitoring and Adjusting Goals

Regularly monitor your progress toward your goals and be willing to adjust them when necessary:

- **Assess Progress:** Evaluate your progress at regular intervals to determine if you're on track.

- **Adjust When Needed:** If you're not making the expected progress, be open to modifying your goals or strategies. It's okay to adjust your timeline or approach.

- **Celebrate Achievements:** Acknowledge and celebrate your accomplishments, even small ones. This reinforces your commitment and keeps you motivated.

- **Seek Guidance:** Consider seeking guidance from fitness professionals or trainers if you're unsure about your goals or progress.

7.9.5: Goal Examples

Here are some examples of muscle-building goals:

- **Increase Strength:** Set specific strength targets for exercises like squats, deadlifts, or bench presses.

- **Improve Endurance:** Work on your cardiovascular fitness to enhance your overall stamina.

- **Nutritional Goals:** Establish dietary goals, such as consuming a certain amount of protein daily or increasing your vegetable intake.

- **Body Composition:** Aim to achieve a particular body fat percentage or gain a specific amount of lean muscle mass.

- **Performance Goals:** Focus on specific performance goals, like running a certain distance in a set time or completing a challenging workout routine.

7.9.6: The Journey Matters

Remember that your muscle-building journey is not solely about reaching the destination but also about the experiences and lessons along the way. Embrace the process, stay adaptable, and continue striving for excellence in your fitness and nutrition.

By setting and adjusting goals effectively, you'll not only enhance your chances of success but also gain a deeper understanding of your capabilities and potential.

7.10. Beyond the Cookbook: Building a Sustainable Lifestyle

Achieving your muscle-building goals is not just about following recipes; it's about adopting a sustainable and balanced lifestyle. In this section, we'll explore how to integrate your muscle-building journey into your daily life, ensuring long-term success and well-being.

7.10.1: Consistency is Key

Consistency is the foundation of a sustainable lifestyle. Here's how to maintain it:

- **Routine:** Establish a consistent workout schedule that fits your life. Make exercise a non-negotiable part of your day.

- **Meal Planning:** Continue using the cookbook's recipes and meal planning strategies to ensure you consistently consume nutritious meals.

7.10.2: Mindful Eating

Practice mindful eating to foster a healthy relationship with food:

- **Savor Your Meals:** Slow down and enjoy the flavors and textures of your food.

- **Listen to Your Body:** Pay attention to hunger and fullness cues, eating when hungry and stopping when satisfied.

- **Avoid Emotional Eating:** Find alternative ways to cope with stress or emotions rather than turning to food.

7.10.3: Balancing Nutrition and Enjoyment

A sustainable lifestyle includes occasional indulgences:

- **Treat Meals:** Allow yourself occasional treat meals to enjoy your favorite foods guilt-free.

- **Balance:** Balance treats with your regular healthy meals and workouts.

7.10.4: Adapt to Life Changes

Life is dynamic, and your muscle-building journey should adapt to changes:

- **Work and Family:** Adjust your routine to accommodate work or family commitments.

- **Travel:** Learn to make nutritious choices while traveling or dining out.

7.10.5: Mental and Emotional Well-Being

Prioritize your mental and emotional health:

- **Stress Management:** Incorporate stress-reduction techniques like meditation, yoga, or hobbies you enjoy.

- **Self-Compassion:** Be kind to yourself. Accept setbacks and mistakes as part of the journey.

7.10.6: Social Support

Involve friends and family in your lifestyle:

- **Workout Partners:** Consider finding a workout partner to motivate each other.

- **Healthy Family Meals:** Encourage nutritious family meals and workouts as a bonding experience.

7.10.7: Continued Learning

Stay informed about fitness and nutrition:

- **Read and Research:** Continuously educate yourself about muscle-building and health-related topics.

- **Experiment:** Be open to trying new workouts, recipes, and techniques to keep things fresh and exciting.

7.10.8: Monitoring and Adjusting

Regularly evaluate your lifestyle and adjust as needed:

- **Progress Tracking:** Continue monitoring your progress and adjust your goals accordingly.

- **Feedback:** Listen to your body and make changes if you experience plateaus or discomfort.

7.10.9: Celebrate Milestones

Acknowledge and celebrate your achievements:

- **Setting New Goals:** Once you achieve a goal, set new ones to keep your journey exciting and purposeful.

- **Reflect:** Take time to reflect on how far you've come and the positive changes you've made.

A sustainable lifestyle extends beyond the recipes in this cookbook. It's about integrating fitness, nutrition, and well-being into your daily life in a way that brings you joy and fulfillment.

By embracing these principles, you'll not only achieve your muscle-building goals but also cultivate a balanced and sustainable lifestyle that enhances your overall quality of life.

APPENDICES

Appendix A: Recommended Reading and Resources

Congratulations on embarking on your muscle-building journey with "Muscle Fuel." To further expand your knowledge and enhance your progress, we've compiled a list of recommended reading materials and online resources. These sources offer valuable insights, expert advice, and a wealth of information to support your fitness and nutrition goals.

Books:

1. "Bigger Leaner Stronger: The Simple Science of Building the Ultimate Male Body" by Michael Matthews

   - A comprehensive guide to strength training, nutrition, and muscle building tailored for men.

2. "Thinner Leaner Stronger: The Simple Science of Building the Ultimate Female Body" by Michael Matthews

   - The female counterpart to the above book, focusing on effective strategies for women's fitness and muscle development.

3. "The New Rules of Lifting for Women" by Lou Schuler and Alwyn Cosgrove

- An empowering resource that challenges common fitness myths and provides practical advice for women looking to build strength and muscle.

4. "Nutrition for Sport and Exercise" by Marie Dunford

- A detailed exploration of sports nutrition principles and strategies to optimize your diet for physical performance.

Websites and Online Resources:

1. **Bodybuilding.com** (www.bodybuilding.com)

- A comprehensive fitness resource featuring workout plans, nutrition articles, and a supportive community of fitness enthusiasts.

2. **MyFitnessPal** (www.myfitnesspal.com)

- A popular app and website for tracking your daily food intake, setting fitness goals, and accessing a vast database of nutritional information.

3. **ExRx.net** (www.exrx.net)

- An invaluable resource for exercise enthusiasts, offering an extensive exercise library, workout plans, and information on muscle anatomy.

4. **PubMed** (www.ncbi.nlm.nih.gov/pubmed)

- Access scientific research articles on nutrition, exercise, and muscle building to stay informed about the latest discoveries in the field.

5. **National Strength and Conditioning Association (NSCA)** (www.nsca.com)

   - The NSCA website provides educational resources, articles, and certifications related to strength and conditioning.

Fitness Apps:

1. **StrongLifts 5x5** (iOS and Android)

   - A popular app for tracking and progressing through strength training workouts.

2. **Fitbod** (iOS and Android)

   - An AI-powered fitness app that creates personalized workout plans based on your goals and equipment availability.

3. **Cronometer** (iOS and Android)

   - A nutrition tracking app that helps you monitor your daily nutrient intake, including protein, vitamins, and minerals.

Podcasts:

1. **The Muscle for Life Podcast** by Michael Matthews

- Michael Matthews, author of "Bigger Leaner Stronger," shares insights on fitness, nutrition, and muscle building.

2. **The Model Health Show** by Shawn Stevenson

- A health and fitness podcast that covers a wide range of topics, including muscle building, nutrition, and holistic wellness.

Remember that knowledge is a powerful tool on your journey to building muscle and improving your overall health. Explore these resources to gain a deeper understanding of the principles discussed in "Muscle Fuel" and to stay motivated and informed as you work toward your goals.

Appendix B: Additional Recipes

In addition to the recipes featured in the main sections of this cookbook, we've curated a selection of extra recipes to add variety to your muscle-building meal plan. These recipes are designed to provide the same balance of nutrients, flavor, and ease of preparation that you've come to expect from "Muscle Fuel." Feel free to incorporate these recipes into your weekly rotation to keep your taste buds excited and your muscles fueled.

B.1. Grilled Lemon Herb Chicken

Ingredients:

- 4 boneless, skinless chicken breasts

- Juice of 1 lemon

- 2 tablespoons olive oil

- 2 cloves garlic, minced

- 1 teaspoon dried oregano

- 1 teaspoon dried thyme

- Salt and black pepper to taste

Instructions:

1. In a bowl, whisk together the lemon juice, olive oil, minced garlic, dried oregano, dried thyme, salt, and black pepper.

2. Place the chicken breasts in a resealable plastic bag or shallow dish and pour the marinade over them.

3. Seal the bag or cover the dish and refrigerate for at least 30 minutes (or up to 24 hours) to marinate.

4. Preheat your grill to medium-high heat.

5. Remove the chicken from the marinade and grill for about 6-8 minutes per side, or until the internal temperature reaches 165°F (74°C).

6. Serve with your choice of steamed vegetables or a fresh salad.

B.2. Quinoa and Black Bean Stuffed Peppers

Ingredients:

- 4 large bell peppers, any color

- 1 cup quinoa, rinsed and drained

- 1 can (15 oz) black beans, drained and rinsed

- 1 cup corn kernels (fresh, frozen, or canned)

- 1 cup diced tomatoes (canned or fresh)

- 1 teaspoon chili powder

- 1/2 teaspoon cumin

- Salt and black pepper to taste

- 1 cup shredded cheddar cheese (optional)

Instructions:

1. Preheat your oven to 375°F (190°C).

2. Cut the tops off the bell peppers and remove the seeds and membranes.

3. In a large saucepan, bring 2 cups of water to a boil. Add the quinoa, reduce heat to low, cover, and simmer for 15 minutes or until quinoa is cooked and water is absorbed.

4. In a large bowl, combine the cooked quinoa, black beans, corn, diced tomatoes, chili powder, cumin, salt, and black pepper.

5. Stuff each bell pepper with the quinoa and black bean mixture.

6. Place the stuffed peppers in a baking dish, cover with aluminum foil, and bake for 25-30 minutes.

7. If desired, remove the foil, sprinkle shredded cheddar cheese on top of each pepper, and bake for an additional 5-7 minutes or until the cheese is melted and bubbly.

B.3. Tropical Protein Smoothie

Ingredients:

- 1 cup unsweetened coconut milk (or your choice of milk)

- 1/2 cup Greek yogurt

- 1 scoop vanilla protein powder

- 1/2 banana

- 1/2 cup pineapple chunks (fresh or frozen)

- 1/2 cup mango chunks (fresh or frozen)

- 1 tablespoon honey (optional)

- Ice cubes (as needed)

Instructions:

1. In a blender, combine the coconut milk, Greek yogurt, vanilla protein powder, banana, pineapple chunks, mango chunks, and honey (if using).

2. Blend until smooth and creamy, adding ice cubes as needed to achieve your desired consistency.

3. Pour into a glass and enjoy this tropical delight as a refreshing post-workout snack or breakfast option.

Feel free to explore these additional recipes to keep your meals interesting and diverse as you work towards your muscle-building goals. Enjoy experimenting with different flavors and ingredients to find your favorite combinations.

Appendix C: Glossary of Terms and Ingredients

This comprehensive index is designed to help you quickly find and understand key terms and ingredients used in "Muscle Fuel: Balanced Recipes for Building Muscles." Whether you're looking for a specific term or want to learn more about an ingredient, this index is your go-to resource.

Terms:

- **Amino Acids:** The building blocks of protein, essential for muscle repair and growth.

- **Carbohydrates:** The body's primary energy source, important for workouts and recovery.

- **Macronutrients:** Nutrients needed in large quantities, including carbohydrates, proteins, and fats.

- **Micronutrients:** Essential vitamins and minerals required in smaller quantities for overall health.

- **Proteins:** Essential for muscle repair and growth, they consist of amino acids.

- **Nutrient Timing:** The strategic timing of meals and nutrients around workouts for optimal performance and recovery.

- **Lean Muscle Mass:** Muscle tissue with minimal fat content.

- **Resistance Training:** Exercise that involves lifting weights or using resistance to build muscle.

- **Body Mass Index (BMI):** A measure of body fat based on height and weight.

- **Lean Body Mass:** Your total weight minus the weight of body fat.

- **Metabolism:** The process by which your body converts food into energy.

- **Calorie Deficit:** Consuming fewer calories than your body needs for weight loss.

- **Calorie Surplus:** Consuming more calories than your body needs for weight gain.

Ingredients:

- **Quinoa:** A high-protein grain that's also a good source of fiber and essential nutrients.

- **Salmon:** A fatty fish rich in omega-3 fatty acids, great for heart health and muscle recovery.

- **Greek Yogurt:** A protein-packed dairy product that's also a source of probiotics.

- **Black Beans:** A protein and fiber-rich legume that's versatile in cooking.

- **Chia Seeds:** Tiny seeds packed with fiber, healthy fats, and essential nutrients.

- **Spinach:** A leafy green vegetable rich in iron and other vitamins and minerals.

- **Lean Beef:** A source of high-quality protein and essential nutrients like iron and zinc.

- **Sweet Potatoes:** A complex carbohydrate source that's rich in vitamins and fiber.

- **Broccoli:** A cruciferous vegetable known for its nutritional value and antioxidants.

- **Almonds:** A nutrient-dense nut rich in healthy fats and protein.

- **Berries:** Fruits like blueberries and strawberries packed with antioxidants.

- **Bananas:** A quick source of natural sugars and potassium for energy.

- **Cottage Cheese:** A dairy product high in protein and low in fat.

- **Peanut Butter:** A spread made from ground peanuts, providing protein and healthy fats.

- **Avocado:** A creamy fruit loaded with healthy fats and vitamins.

- **Dates:** Sweet fruits high in natural sugars and fiber.

- **Lemon-Dill Sauce:** A flavorful sauce made with lemon juice and fresh dill.

- **Cumin:** A spice with a warm, earthy flavor often used in savory dishes.

- **Chili Powder:** A blend of spices, including chili peppers and cumin, for adding heat and flavor.

Appendix D: Cooking Techniques

In "Muscle Fuel," we want to empower you with not only delicious recipes but also the knowledge and skills to master various cooking techniques. This appendix serves as a guide to the fundamental cooking methods and tips you'll encounter throughout the cookbook, ensuring your meals are not only nutritious but also bursting with flavor.

D.1. Grilling

Grilling is a fantastic way to add a smoky, charred flavor to your dishes while keeping them lean and healthy. Here are some grilling tips:

- **Preheat the Grill:** Ensure your grill is hot before placing food on it. Preheating prevents sticking and helps sear the food.

- **Oil the Grill Grates:** Brush oil on the grates before grilling to prevent sticking.

- **Marinate for Flavor:** Marinating meats and vegetables adds flavor and tenderizes them.

- **Direct vs. Indirect Heat:** Learn when to use direct heat (for searing) and indirect heat (for slow cooking) on your grill.

D.2. Roasting

Roasting involves cooking food in the oven at high temperatures, creating a crispy exterior and preserving moisture. Key roasting tips:

- **Preheat the Oven:** Ensure the oven is at the right temperature before placing food inside.

- **Use a Roasting Pan:** A roasting pan with a rack allows air circulation for even cooking.

- **Season Well:** Season food with herbs, spices, and a drizzle of oil for added flavor.

- **Check Doneness:** Use a meat thermometer to check the internal temperature of meats.

D.3. Sautéing

Sautéing is a quick-cooking method in a pan with a small amount of oil. Tips for successful sautéing:

- **Hot Pan:** Use a hot pan to cook ingredients quickly without overcrowding the pan.

- **Uniform Size:** Cut ingredients into uniform sizes for even cooking.

- **Stir Frequently:** Stirring prevents sticking and ensures even cooking.

- **Finish with Sauce:** Deglaze the pan with broth, wine, or sauce to create a flavorful finish.

D.4. Blending and Pureeing

Blending and pureeing create smooth textures and combine ingredients into delicious sauces, smoothies, and soups:

- **Blender vs. Food Processor:** Choose the right appliance based on the consistency you desire.

- **Start Slow:** When blending hot liquids, start at a low speed to prevent splattering.

- **Taste and Adjust:** Blend, taste, and adjust seasonings to your preference.

D.5. Steaming

Steaming is a healthy cooking method that preserves nutrients and flavors:

- **Use a Steamer Basket:** Place ingredients in a steamer basket over boiling water.

- **Cover Tightly:** Steam food with a tight-fitting lid to trap steam and cook evenly.

- **Quick Cool:** To stop cooking, transfer steamed food to an ice bath.

D.6. Baking

Baking is ideal for preparing casseroles, baked goods, and dishes with a golden-brown crust:

- **Preheat the Oven:** Ensure the oven is fully preheated for consistent results.

- **Use Baking Pans:** Choose appropriate bakeware and follow suggested temperatures and times.

- **Rotate Dishes:** Rotate pans during baking for even cooking.

These fundamental cooking techniques will serve you well as you explore the recipes in "Muscle Fuel." Don't hesitate to experiment and develop your culinary skills, adding your unique touch to each dish. Happy cooking!

Appendix E: Sample Meal Plans

To simplify your journey toward building muscle and maintaining a balanced diet, we've prepared these sample meal plans. Each plan includes a combination of recipes from "Muscle Fuel," ensuring you receive a variety of nutrients while enjoying delicious meals throughout the day. Feel free to use these plans as a starting point, adjusting portion sizes and ingredients to suit your individual needs and preferences.

E.1. Meal Plan: Balanced Muscle Builder

Breakfast:

- **1.1. Protein-Packed Oatmeal**

- 1 serving of mixed berries

- A handful of almonds

Lunch:

- **2.3. Turkey and Veggie Wrap**

- A side of raw baby carrots and cucumber slices

Snack:

- **4.1. Protein-Packed Smoothie**

- 1 banana

- 1 tablespoon of almond butter

Dinner:

- **3.5. Roasted Vegetable Quinoa Bowl**

- Grilled chicken breast (optional)

- A side salad with vinaigrette dressing

Snack:

- 1 serving of Greek yogurt with honey

E.2. Meal Plan: Vegetarian Muscle Fuel

Breakfast:

- **1.3. Greek Yogurt Parfait**

- Mixed with chia seeds and topped with fresh berries

Lunch:

- **2.2. Chickpea and Spinach Salad**

- Served with a whole-grain roll

Snack:

- A small handful of mixed nuts

Dinner:

- **3.4. Citrus-Marinated Grilled Chicken**

- Steamed broccoli

- Quinoa

Snack:

- **4.2. Almond and Dark Chocolate Energy Bites**

E.3. Meal Plan: High Protein Power

Breakfast:

- **1.5. High-Protein Pancakes**

- Topped with Greek yogurt and a drizzle of honey

Lunch:

- **2.5. Mediterranean Power Plate**

- A side of whole-grain pita bread

Snack:

- A protein shake with your favorite protein powder

Dinner:

- **3.1. Baked Salmon with Lemon-Dill Sauce**

- Asparagus spears

- Quinoa

Snack:

- **5.5. Greek Yogurt Berry Parfait**

These sample meal plans are designed to help you maintain a balanced diet while supporting your muscle-building goals. Adjust portion sizes and ingredients as needed to meet your specific calorie and nutrient requirements. Feel free to mix and match recipes to create your customized meal plans based on your preferences and dietary needs.

Remember, the key to success is consistency and a well-rounded approach to nutrition. Enjoy your journey towards building a stronger, healthier you!

Appendix F: Workout Plans

A successful muscle-building journey doesn't rely solely on nutrition; it also requires a well-structured workout plan. This appendix presents sample workout plans suitable for various fitness levels. Remember to consult with a fitness professional before starting any new exercise program, especially if you have underlying health conditions.

F.1. Beginner's Muscle-Building Workout

Day 1: Full-Body Workout

- Squats: 3 sets of 10 reps

- Push-Ups (knee or regular): 3 sets of 10 reps

- Bent-Over Dumbbell Rows: 3 sets of 10 reps

- Plank: 3 sets of 30 seconds

Day 2: Rest

Day 3: Full-Body Workout

- Lunges: 3 sets of 10 reps per leg

- Dumbbell Bench Press (on the floor or a bench): 3 sets of 10 reps

- Bicep Curls: 3 sets of 10 reps

- Bicycle Crunches: 3 sets of 15 reps per side

Day 4: Rest

Day 5: Full-Body Workout

- Deadlift (use light weights or a barbell): 3 sets of 10 reps

- Lat Pulldowns (using a resistance band or machine): 3 sets of 10 reps

- Tricep Dips (use parallel bars or a sturdy chair): 3 sets of 10 reps

- Leg Raises: 3 sets of 12 reps

Day 6 and 7: Rest

F.2. Intermediate Muscle-Building Workout

Day 1: Upper Body

- Bench Press: 3 sets of 8-10 reps

- Pull-Ups or Lat Pulldowns: 3 sets of 8-10 reps

- Dumbbell Rows: 3 sets of 10 reps per arm

- Push-Ups: 3 sets of 10-12 reps

- Plank: 3 sets of 45 seconds

Day 2: Lower Body

- Squats: 3 sets of 8-10 reps

- Deadlifts: 3 sets of 8-10 reps

- Lunges: 3 sets of 10 reps per leg

- Leg Press: 3 sets of 10-12 reps

- Russian Twists: 3 sets of 12 reps per side

Day 3: Rest

Day 4: Full-Body

- Incline Bench Press: 3 sets of 8-10 reps

- Pull-Ups or Lat Pulldowns: 3 sets of 8-10 reps

- Barbell Rows: 3 sets of 10 reps

- Dumbbell Shoulder Press: 3 sets of 10-12 reps

- Plank: 3 sets of 45 seconds

Day 5: Rest

Day 6: Full-Body

- Sumo Deadlift: 3 sets of 8-10 reps

- Pull-Ups or Lat Pulldowns: 3 sets of 8-10 reps

- Tricep Dips: 3 sets of 10 reps

- Leg Raises: 3 sets of 12 reps

- Bicycle Crunches: 3 sets of 15 reps per side

Day 7: Rest

F.3. Advanced Muscle-Building Workout

Day 1: Chest and Triceps

- Bench Press: 4 sets of 8-10 reps

- Incline Dumbbell Press: 4 sets of 8-10 reps

- Tricep Dips: 4 sets of 8-10 reps

- Skull Crushers: 4 sets of 8-10 reps

Day 2: Back and Biceps

- Deadlifts: 4 sets of 6-8 reps

- Pull-Ups or Lat Pulldowns: 4 sets of 8-10 reps

- Barbell Rows: 4 sets of 8-10 reps

- Barbell Bicep Curls: 4 sets of 8-10 reps

Day 3: Rest

Day 4: Shoulders and Abs

- Overhead Shoulder Press: 4 sets of 8-10 reps

- Lateral Raises: 4 sets of 10-12 reps

- Front Raises: 4 sets of 10-12 reps

- Hanging Leg Raises: 4 sets of 12-15 reps

- Russian Twists: 4 sets of 15 reps per side

Day 5: Legs

- Squats: 4 sets of 8-10 reps

- Lunges: 4 sets of 8-10 reps per leg

- Leg Press: 4 sets of 10-12 reps

- Romanian Deadlifts: 4 sets of 8-10 reps

Day 6 and 7: Rest

These workout plans provide a structured approach to strength training. Remember to warm up before each session and cool down afterward. Gradually increase weights and repetitions as you progress in your fitness journey. Additionally, always prioritize proper form and technique to prevent injury.

Appendix G: Frequently Asked Questions (FAQ)

We understand that embarking on a muscle-building journey and exploring a new cookbook can lead to questions. Below, we've compiled answers to some of the most frequently asked questions to support your journey with "Muscle Fuel."

G.1. Nutrition and Diet Questions

Q1. What's the importance of nutrition in muscle building? A1. Nutrition plays a pivotal role in muscle building. Consuming the right balance of macronutrients (protein, carbohydrates, and fats) and micronutrients (vitamins and minerals) provides the necessary fuel and building blocks for muscle growth and recovery.

Q2. How many calories should I consume daily for muscle building? A2. Caloric needs vary based on factors like age, gender, activity level, and goals. Generally, a slight calorie surplus (more calories in than burned) is needed for muscle gain, but it should be personalized to your needs.

Q3. Can I build muscle on a vegetarian or vegan diet? A3. Absolutely! Many plant-based protein sources like beans, lentils, tofu, and quinoa can support muscle growth. Ensure you include a variety of protein-rich foods to meet your needs.

Q4. Do I need supplements for muscle building? A4. Whole foods should be your primary source of nutrients. However, some individuals may benefit from supplements like protein powder, creatine, or branched-chain amino acids (BCAAs). Consult a healthcare professional before using supplements.

G.2. Cookbook and Recipe Questions

Q5. Can I adjust the portion sizes in the recipes? A5. Certainly! Feel free to adjust portion sizes to match your dietary goals and needs. The recipes are flexible, and you can customize them to your preferences.

Q6. Can I substitute ingredients in the recipes? A6. Absolutely. Substitutions can be made to accommodate dietary preferences or allergies. Just be mindful that ingredient substitutions may affect the nutritional content and flavor of the dish.

Q7. Are the recipes suitable for meal prep? A7. Yes, many of the recipes in "Muscle Fuel" are great for meal prep. Prepare larger batches and portion them into containers for convenient, ready-to-eat meals throughout the week.

Q8. Can I use these recipes for weight loss? A8. While the focus of the cookbook is on muscle building, you can adapt the recipes for weight loss by adjusting portion sizes and ensuring you maintain a caloric deficit.

G.3. Muscle-Building and Fitness Questions

Q9. How often should I work out to build muscle? A9. Consistency is key. Aim for at least three to four days of strength training per week, targeting different muscle groups. Allow time for rest and recovery as well.

Q10. Can I build muscle without lifting heavy weights? A10. Yes, resistance training can involve various levels of resistance, including bodyweight exercises, resistance bands, and lighter weights. The key is progressive overload—gradually increasing resistance over time.

Q11. What's the importance of rest and recovery in muscle building?
A11. Rest and recovery are essential for muscle repair and growth. Overtraining can lead to injury and hinder progress. Ensure you get enough sleep and incorporate rest days into your workout routine.

These FAQs are here to provide clarity and guidance on your muscle-building journey with "Muscle Fuel." If you have additional questions or need personalized advice, don't hesitate to seek support from a healthcare professional or fitness expert.

Appendix H: Tracking Tools and Templates

Tracking your nutrition, workouts, and progress is crucial in achieving your muscle-building goals. In this appendix, we've provided useful tools and templates to assist you on your journey with "Muscle Fuel."

H.1. Meal Planning Template

Meal Planning Template

Date: ______________

Breakfast:

- ✓ Recipe name

- ✓ Ingredients needed

- ✓ Preparation steps

Lunch:

- ✓ ☒ Recipe name
- ✓ ☒ Ingredients needed
- ✓ ☒ Preparation steps

Snack:

- ✓ ☒ Recipe name
- ✓ ☒ Ingredients needed
- ✓ ☒ Preparation steps

Dinner:

- ✓ ☒ Recipe name
- ✓ ☒ Ingredients needed
- ✓ ☒ Preparation steps

Snack:

- ✓ ☒ Recipe name
- ✓ ☒ Ingredients needed
- ✓ ☒ Preparation steps

Use this meal planning template to organize your daily meals and ensure you're incorporating a variety of recipes from "Muscle Fuel" into your diet.

H.2. Workout Log

Workout Log

Date: _______________

Exercise:

- ✓ ☒ Exercise name
- ✓ ☒ Sets
- ✓ ☒ Repetitions
- ✓ ☒ Weight/Resistance
- ✓ ☒ Notes/Progress

Exercise:

- ✓ ☒ Exercise name
- ✓ ☒ Sets
- ✓ ☒ Repetitions
- ✓ ☒ Weight/Resistance

- ✓ ☒ Notes/Progress

Exercise:

- ✓ ☒ Exercise name

- ✓ ☒ Sets

- ✓ ☒ Repetitions

- ✓ ☒ Weight/Resistance

- ✓ ☒ Notes/Progress

Use this workout log to track your strength training sessions, including the exercises, sets, repetitions, and any notes on your progress or adjustments.

H.3. Progress Tracker

Progress Tracker

Date: _______________

Measurements:

- ✓ ☒ Weight

- ✓ ☒ Body Measurements (chest, waist, hips, etc.)

- ✓ ☒ Body Fat Percentage (if available)

Nutrition:

- ✓ ☒ Daily Caloric Intake
- ✓ ☒ Protein Intake
- ✓ ☒ Carbohydrate Intake
- ✓ ☒ Fat Intake

Fitness:

- ✓ ☒ Strength Progress (e.g., increased weight lifted)
- ✓ ☒ Endurance Progress (e.g., longer workout duration)
- ✓ ☒ Any Achieved Fitness Goals (e.g., completed a 5k run)

Use this progress tracker to record your measurements, nutrition data, and fitness achievements over time. Regularly updating it can help you stay motivated and track your muscle-building journey.

H.4. Shopping List Template

Shopping List Template

Date: _______________

Proteins:

- ✓ ☒ List of protein sources and quantities needed

Carbohydrates:

- ✓ ☒ List of carbohydrate sources and quantities needed

Fats:

- ✓ ☒ List of fat sources and quantities needed

Produce:

- ✓ ☒ List of fruits and vegetables needed

Dairy/Alternatives:

- ✓ ☒ List of dairy or dairy alternatives needed

Pantry Staples:

- ✓ ☒ List of spices, condiments, and other pantry items needed

Use this shopping list template to plan your grocery trips efficiently, ensuring you have all the ingredients you need for your muscle-building recipes.

These tracking tools and templates are designed to help you stay organized, monitor your progress, and make informed choices throughout your muscle-building journey. Customize and use them as needed to support your individual goals and preferences.

Appendix I: Shopping Lists

To help you prepare the delicious recipes in "Muscle Fuel" with ease, we've created comprehensive shopping lists for each section of the cookbook. These lists outline the ingredients you'll need to stock up on, ensuring your kitchen is well-prepared for your muscle-building journey.

I.1. Breakfast Boosters

- ✓ Rolled oats
- ✓ Greek yogurt
- ✓ Eggs
- ✓ Spinach
- ✓ Feta cheese
- ✓ Whole wheat flour
- ✓ Protein powder (optional)
- ✓ Almond milk
- ✓ Bananas
- ✓ Almonds
- ✓ Mixed berries

- ✓ ☒ Honey

- ✓ ☒ Olive oil

- ✓ ☒ Salt and pepper

I.2. Lunchtime Power Plates

- ✓ ☒ Chicken breast or thigh fillets

- ✓ ☒ Quinoa

- ✓ ☒ Chickpeas

- ✓ ☒ Spinach

- ✓ ☒ Cherry tomatoes

- ✓ ☒ Red onion

- ✓ ☒ Feta cheese

- ✓ ☒ Olive oil

- ✓ ☒ Balsamic vinegar

- ✓ ☒ Salt and pepper

- ✓ ☒ Whole wheat tortillas

- ✓ ☒ Turkey slices

- ✓ ☒ Hummus
- ✓ ☒ Cucumber
- ✓ ☒ Red bell pepper
- ✓ ☒ Salmon fillets
- ✓ ☒ Asparagus
- ✓ ☒ Lemon
- ✓ ☒ Oregano
- ✓ ☒ Garlic
- ✓ ☒ Brown rice
- ✓ ☒ Zucchini
- ✓ ☒ Yellow squash
- ✓ ☒ Red bell pepper
- ✓ ☒ Red onion
- ✓ ☒ Olive oil
- ✓ ☒ Paprika
- ✓ ☒ Cumin

- Ground coriander

- Dried oregano

- Black beans

- Sweet potatoes

- Ground beef or turkey

- Onion

- Garlic

- Taco seasoning

- Spinach

- Eggs

- Feta cheese

- Olive oil

- Salt and pepper

I.3. Dinner Delights

- Salmon fillets

- Lemon

✓ ☒ Dill

✓ ☒ Olive oil

✓ ☒ Salt and pepper

✓ ☒ Lean beef (e.g., sirloin or tenderloin)

✓ ☒ Soy sauce

✓ ☒ Honey

✓ ☒ Garlic

✓ ☒ Ginger

✓ ☒ Broccoli

✓ ☒ Red bell pepper

✓ ☒ Onion

✓ ☒ Red kidney beans

✓ ☒ Black beans

✓ ☒ Diced tomatoes

✓ ☒ Chili powder

✓ ☒ Ground cumin

- ✓ ☒ Paprika

- ✓ ☒ Cayenne pepper

- ✓ ☒ Olive oil

- ✓ ☒ Chicken breasts

- ✓ ☒ Orange juice

- ✓ ☒ Lemon juice

- ✓ ☒ Garlic

- ✓ ☒ Rosemary

- ✓ ☒ Dijon mustard

- ✓ ☒ Mixed vegetables (e.g., bell peppers, zucchini, carrots)

- ✓ ☒ Quinoa

- ✓ ☒ Olive oil

- ✓ ☒ Salt and pepper

I.4. Snacks for Strength

- ✓ ☒ Protein powder

- ✓ ☒ Almond milk

- ☑ Almonds

- ☑ Dark chocolate chips

- ☑ Cottage cheese

- ☑ Mixed berries

- ☑ Hummus

- ☑ Carrot sticks

- ☑ Celery sticks

- ☑ Cucumber slices

- ☑ Nut butter (e.g., almond or peanut)

- ☑ Whole grain bread or toast

I.5. Desserts with a Twist

- ☑ Avocado

- ☑ Cocoa powder

- ☑ Maple syrup

- ☑ Vanilla extract

- ☑ Greek yogurt

- ✓ ☒ Apples

- ✓ ☒ Cinnamon

- ✓ ☒ Mixed berries

- ✓ ☒ Protein powder

- ✓ ☒ Peanut butter

- ✓ ☒ Dates

- ✓ ☒ Almonds

- ✓ ☒ Dark chocolate chips

I.6. Sides and Extras

- ✓ ☒ Quinoa

- ✓ ☒ Black beans

- ✓ ☒ Corn

- ✓ ☒ Red bell pepper

- ✓ ☒ Fresh cilantro

- ✓ ☒ Lime juice

- ✓ ☒ Olive oil

- ✓ ☒ Garlic

- ✓ ☒ Salt and pepper

- ✓ ☒ Broccoli

- ✓ ☒ Garlic

- ✓ ☒ Olive oil

- ✓ ☒ Salt and pepper

- ✓ ☒ Sweet potatoes

- ✓ ☒ Olive oil

- ✓ ☒ Paprika

- ✓ ☒ Spinach

- ✓ ☒ Feta cheese

- ✓ ☒ Mushrooms

- ✓ ☒ Garlic

- ✓ ☒ Olive oil

- ✓ ☒ Asparagus

- ✓ ☒ Lemon

✓ ☒ Olive oil

Use these shopping lists to streamline your grocery shopping trips and ensure you have all the necessary ingredients on hand to create the delectable muscle-building recipes from "Muscle Fuel."

Appendix J: Conversion Charts

In the kitchen, precise measurements are essential to achieving the perfect results in your recipes. These conversion charts will help you switch between various units of measurement effortlessly, ensuring your cooking and baking endeavors in "Muscle Fuel" are a breeze.

J.1. Volume Conversion Chart

- 1 teaspoon (tsp) = 5 milliliters (ml)

- 1 tablespoon (tbsp) = 15 milliliters (ml)

- 1 fluid ounce (fl oz) = 30 milliliters (ml)

- 1 cup (c) = 240 milliliters (ml)

- 1 pint (pt) = 480 milliliters (ml)

- 1 quart (qt) = 960 milliliters (ml)

- 1 liter (l) = 1,000 milliliters (ml)

- 1 gallon (gal) = 3,840 milliliters (ml)

J.2. Weight Conversion Chart

- 1 ounce (oz) = 28 grams (g)

- 1 pound (lb) = 453 grams (g)

- 1 kilogram (kg) = 1,000 grams (g)

J.3. Temperature Conversion Chart

- Celsius (°C) to Fahrenheit (°F):

    - $[°F] = ([°C] \times 9/5) + 32$

- Fahrenheit (°F) to Celsius (°C):

    - $[°C] = ([°F] - 32) \times 5/9$

J.4. Common Ingredient Equivalents

- 1 egg = 1/4 cup applesauce (as a vegan substitute)

- 1 cup buttermilk = 1 cup milk + 1 tablespoon white vinegar or lemon juice (let sit for 5 minutes)

- 1 cup sour cream = 1 cup Greek yogurt (for a healthier option)

- 1 cup breadcrumbs = 1 cup crushed crackers or panko breadcrumbs

- 1 cup granulated sugar = 1 cup brown sugar (for a richer flavor)

- 1 stick of butter = 1/2 cup (8 tablespoons)

J.5. Pan Size Conversion

- 9-inch round cake pan = 8-inch square cake pan

- 9x13-inch baking dish = 2 (9-inch) round cake pans

- 9x13-inch baking dish = 3 (8-inch) round cake pans

These conversion charts will assist you in adapting the recipes in "Muscle Fuel" to suit your preferred units of measurement and ingredient substitutions. Happy cooking!

Appendix K: Nutritional Information

Understanding the nutritional content of your meals is crucial for achieving your muscle-building goals. This appendix provides the key nutritional information for the recipes featured in "Muscle Fuel."

K.1. Nutritional Information Guide

- **Calories:** The total energy content of one serving.

- **Protein:** The amount of protein in one serving, a vital nutrient for muscle growth and repair.

- **Carbohydrates:** The total carbohydrates, including dietary fiber and sugars, in one serving.

- **Dietary Fiber:** The portion of carbohydrates that is indigestible and important for digestive health.

- **Sugars:** The natural or added sugars present in one serving.

- **Total Fat:** The total fat content, which includes saturated and unsaturated fats.

- **Saturated Fat:** The portion of total fat that is saturated, which should be consumed in moderation.

- **Trans Fat:** The amount of trans fats, which should be minimized in a healthy diet.

- **Cholesterol:** The cholesterol content per serving.

- **Sodium:** The sodium content, which affects overall health and should be monitored.

- **Vitamins and Minerals:** Information on specific vitamins and minerals, including vitamin A, vitamin C, calcium, and iron.

- **% Daily Value:** The percentage of the daily recommended intake based on a 2,000-calorie diet.

K.2. Recipe Nutritional Information

Please note that the nutritional information provided is approximate and can vary depending on ingredient brands and portion sizes.

Recipe Title: [Name of the Recipe]

- **Calories:** [Number of Calories]

- **Protein:** [Amount of Protein] grams

- **Carbohydrates:** [Amount of Carbohydrates] grams

- **Dietary Fiber:** [Amount of Dietary Fiber] grams

- **Sugars:** [Amount of Sugars] grams

- **Total Fat:** [Amount of Total Fat] grams

- **Saturated Fat:** [Amount of Saturated Fat] grams

- **Trans Fat:** [Amount of Trans Fat] grams

- **Cholesterol:** [Amount of Cholesterol] milligrams

- **Sodium:** [Amount of Sodium] milligrams

- **Vitamin A:** [Amount of Vitamin A] micrograms (or International Units, IU)

- **Vitamin C:** [Amount of Vitamin C] milligrams

- **Calcium:** [Amount of Calcium] milligrams

- **Iron:** [Amount of Iron] milligrams

- **% Daily Value:**

  - Vitamin A: [Percentage of Daily Value]

  - Vitamin C: [Percentage of Daily Value]

  - Calcium: [Percentage of Daily Value]

  - Iron: [Percentage of Daily Value]

Use this nutritional information to make informed dietary choices and track your nutrient intake as you follow the recipes in "Muscle Fuel."

Appendix L: Recipe Index

Breakfast Boosters

1. Protein-Packed Oatmeal

2. Muscle-Building Breakfast Burrito

3. Greek Yogurt Parfait

4. Scrambled Eggs with Spinach and Feta

5. High-Protein Pancakes

Lunchtime Power Plates

6. Grilled Chicken Quinoa Bowl

7. Chickpea and Spinach Salad

8. Turkey and Veggie Wrap

9. Salmon and Asparagus Foil Pack

10. Mediterranean Power Plate

11. Veggie-Packed Quinoa Stuffed Peppers

12. Tofu and Broccoli Stir-Fry

13. Sweet Potato and Black Bean Bowl

14. Spinach and Mushroom Frittata

15.   Beef and Broccoli Rice Bowl

Dinner Delights

16.   Baked Salmon with Lemon-Dill Sauce

17.   Lean Beef Stir-Fry

18.   Vegetarian Chili with Beans

19.   Citrus-Marinated Grilled Chicken

20.   Roasted Vegetable Quinoa Bowl

Snacks for Strength

21.   Protein-Packed Smoothie

22.   Almond and Dark Chocolate Energy Bites

23.   Cottage Cheese and Berries

24.   Hummus and Veggie Platter

25.   Nut Butter Banana Toast

Desserts with a Twist

26.   Protein-Packed Chocolate Avocado Mousse

27.   Baked Apple with Greek Yogurt and Cinnamon

28.   Protein-Packed Fruit Salad

29.   Peanut Butter Banana Ice Cream

30.   Greek Yogurt Berry Parfait

31.   Chocolate Protein Bites

32.   Protein-Packed Rice Pudding

33.   Almond and Date Protein Bars

34.   Chocolate Protein Pancakes

35.   Protein-Rich Chia Pudding

Sides and Extras

36.   Quinoa and Black Bean Salad

37.   Garlic Roasted Broccoli

38.   Sweet Potato Fries

39.   Spinach and Feta Stuffed Mushrooms

40.   Grilled Asparagus with Lemon